MW01113947

MISCARRIAGE

A
*W*OMAN
DOCTOR'S
GUIDE

BOOK YOUR PLACE ON OUR WEBSITE AND MAKE THE READING CONNECTION!

We've created a customized website just for our very special readers, where you can get the inside scoop on everything that's going on with Zebra, Pinnacle and Kensington books.

When you come online, you'll have the exciting opportunity to:

- View covers of upcoming books
- Read sample chapters
- Learn about our future publishing schedule (listed by publication month *and author*)
- Find out when your favorite authors will be visiting a city near you
- Search for and order backlist books from our online catalog
- Check out author bios and background information
- Send e-mail to your favorite authors
- Meet the Kensington staff online
- Join us in weekly chats with authors, readers and other guests
- Get writing guidelines
- AND MUCH MORE!

Visit our website at
http://www.kensingtonbooks.com

MISCARRIAGE

A *WOMAN* DOCTOR'S GUIDE

The Support and Facts You Need to Get Through Pregnancy Loss

LYNN FRIEDMAN, M.D.

with Irene Daria

KENSINGTON BOOKS
KENSINGTON PUBLISHING CORP.
hhtp://www.kensingtonbooks.com

KENSINGTON BOOKS are published by

Kensington Publishing Corp.
850 Third Avenue
New York, NY 10022

Copyright © 1996, 2001 by Lowenstein Associates
Illustrations copyright © 1996 by Mona Mark

All rights reserved. No part of this book may be reproduced in any form or by any means without the prior written consent of the Publisher, excepting brief quotes used in reviews.

All Kensington titles, imprints and distributed lines are available at special quantity discounts for bulk purchases for sales promotion, premiums, fund raising, educational or institutional use.

Special book excerpts or customized printings can also be created to fit specific needs. For details, write or phone the office of the Kensington Special Sales Manager: Kensington Publishing Corp., 850 Third Avenue, New York, NY, 10022. Attn. Special Sales Department. Phone: 1-800-221-2647.

If you purchased this book without a cover you should be aware that this book is stolen property. It was reported as "unsold and destroyed" to the Publisher and neither the Author nor the Publisher has received any payment for this "stripped book."

Kensington and the K logo Reg. U.S. Pat. & TM Off.

First Kensington Paperback Printing: March, 2001
10 9 8 7 6 5 4 3 2 1

Printed in the United States of America

To my husband Ricky and sons Josh and Jake,
the three greatest living beings on earth!
I love you guys!
—Dr. Lynn Friedman

To Peanut,
Your brief existence brought us so much joy, and your
death caused us so much pain. You changed our lives
in so many positive and permanent ways. Writing
this book helped me come to understand why we lost
you. Now, your memory is resting in peace.
—Irene Daria

▼
CONTENTS

▼
LIST OF
ILLUSTRATIONS

INTRODUCTION

Every year, approximately five million women in the United States become pregnant and immediately begin to experience the wonderful hopes and dreams that come with expecting a child. For at least one million of these women, however, these hopes and dreams will end in heartbreak because, according to the most often quoted and most conservative statistics, about 20 percent of all pregnancies end in miscarriage.

The real miscarriage rate, however, is believed to be closer to 40 or 50 percent. This figure cannot be more accurately documented since women often miscarry before they even know they are pregnant; in these cases, they think their miscarriages are simply late, heavy periods. In fact, some women who believe they are infertile are actually conceiving, but are repeatedly miscarrying.

The term *miscarriage* refers to the loss of a developing pregnancy at any time from conception until the twentieth week after the last menstrual period. (After the twentieth week, that loss is considered a death in utero.) All miscarriages fall into one of two categories:

1. *Isolated.* This means they were just that—a chance event often due to a nonrecurring chromosomal error in the egg or sperm or other sporadic event.
2. *Recurring.* After suffering three consecutive miscarriages, a woman becomes classified as a habitual or recurrent aborter. (Many women take offense at the word "abortion" being used to describe a miscarriage, since the term is commonly used to refer to an elective procedure a woman undergoes to terminate an unwanted pregnancy. In medical terminology, however, abortion simply refers to the loss of a pregnancy with no implication of its being a loss by choice.)

Women classified as habitual or recurrent aborters repeatedly miscarry due to some underlying condition that will generally need to be treated before they are able to carry to term. Twenty percent of the women who miscarry become recurrent aborters.

Miscarriage is one of the most medically simple, yet psychologically complex, events that can happen to a woman. Medically, it isn't life threatening to the mother. Pain and blood loss are usually minimal, physical recovery is quick, and the woman's day-to-day physical functioning is not impaired.

Psychologically, however, a miscarriage can be devastating because it involves the death of a child—a child the woman will never get to see, yet may have already grown to love. When a woman mourns for her lost child, she is actually mourning a dream—a vision of what her child would have been—as opposed to mourning a living being she has gotten to know. This fact makes her grieving extraordinarily complex, and this complexity is made worse by the fact that so many women don't talk about their miscarriages. Those who want to are often inhibited by their husbands, friends, and relatives, who often become obviously uncomfortable whenever the women try to raise the subject. At a time when she needs her loved ones most, a woman who has miscarried often ends up feeling unsupported and abandoned.

It's quite odd that a society as open as ours still keeps miscarriage under wraps. Some women embrace that secrecy, relieved that they don't have to answer a barrage of questions about what went wrong. Others are hurt by the silence. They begin to feel that something shameful has happened to them, something they, for some reason, *shouldn't* talk about. Their inability to mourn openly causes their grief to fester and linger longer than it otherwise would.

Since you've picked up this book, chances are you've suffered a miscarriage, and you've probably experienced that odd shroud of silence that surrounds it. With this book I would like to shatter some of that silence and explain why your loss occurred, whether you've just suffered your first miscarriage or whether you've had two, three, four, or more. I would also like to reassure you that miscarriage is extremely common and that most women who have miscarriages go on to have healthy babies.

In the following pages, I will cover the most common causes of miscarriage, offer advice on how to handle your physical loss and your emotional pain, and tell you how you can determine when you're ready to conceive again.

1

▼

FACT VS. FICTION

During the entire course of human history, myths have been created when facts were either unavailable or hard to come by. The same holds true for the many myths surrounding miscarriage. Because women who have had miscarriages tend not to talk about them, women in general have no idea how common they really are. Also, because women don't make it known how deeply their miscarriages affect them, and how desperately they need information on the subject, the media tends to ignore the issue. It is astonishing how few books and magazine articles exist on an emotionally wrenching experience that one million women endure every year.

Doctors, on the other hand, treat women for miscarriages on an almost daily basis, and often become immune to what a devastating ordeal it can be. They tend to take care of the medical crisis and then send women on their way with little information as to why they may have miscarried or on how to handle it.

Most women are desperate to know why they have miscarried. This feeling is understandable; it is human nature to try to understand the reasons why bad things happen. Unfortunately, when women wonder why they've miscarried and don't get answers from either their doctors or the media, they turn to hearsay for answers, answers that are often wrong. Not knowing that what they've heard is incorrect, they accept it as truth, causing the myths to spread.

Most of these myths deal with what causes miscarriage, and these are the most worrisome. They cause women to believe they did something wrong, such as lifting a heavy box or taking an airplane trip. Women then blame themselves for their miscarriages, which is a terrible burden to carry, especially since miscarriage usually has nothing to do with what a woman has done.

For this reason, it's important to begin by dispelling some of the most common myths:

Myth #1 Once you've miscarried, you will never be able to carry to term, or you will have tremendous difficulty doing so.

Single miscarriages are extremely common, accounting for 80 percent of all miscarriages. The vast majority of women with an isolated miscarriage can expect to have normal reproductive function with their next pregnancy.

Myth #2 It's "natures way," and there's nothing you can do about it but keep on trying to have a baby.

Twenty percent of the time, an underlying physical condition will cause women to miscarry repeatedly. After treatment, these women go on to have successful pregnancies 70 to 80 percent of the time.

Doctors used to wait until a woman suffered three consecutive miscarriages before testing for underlying problems. Now, with so many women conceiving later in life, doctors will often recommend tests after two *consecutive* miscarriages. (If you have a child between two miscarriages the chance of your having an underlying condition that's causing you to miscarry is less likely.)

Myth #3 It's no big deal.

Most women who miscarry experience significant grief. Miscarriage can affect everything from a woman's self-esteem to her friendships and her marriage. It's important for women to know that mourning is normal and is to be expected. It's equally important for their doctors to be aware of the extent of their grief. Recent research has found that the more sensitive health-care professionals are, the shorter the woman's period of bereavement. It follows that the shorter her period of grief, the sooner she'll be emotionally ready to try to conceive again.

Myth #4 Miscarriages occur most often in first pregnancies.

Because women attach so much more importance to a miscarriage that happens with their first pregnancy—since they don't yet know if they will ever be able to carry to term—it may seem that they occur more frequently at that time. There are no statistics that support this conclusion. In fact, women are more likely to miscarry in subsequent pregnancies. This is the case because by the time many women today become pregnant with their second or third child, they're over age 35. After that, the miscarriage rates are higher simply because the chance of chromosomal problems occurring is greater.

Myth #5 *If you've had one elective abortion, your chance of miscarrying is greater.*

Women who have had fewer than four to five elective first-trimester abortions are not assumed to have any increased risk of miscarrying their subsequent pregnancies. An elective abortion is performed by mechanically opening the cervix and removing the pregnancy tissue. Performing this mechanical dilatation more than four to five times may be linked to an increased rate of miscarriage due to weakening of the cervix. However, women from Eastern European countries whose only available method of birth control is pregnancy termination often have as many as ten or twelve first-trimester abortions. Eventually, when these women want to carry to term, most have no problem doing so.

Second-trimester abortions can affect one's ability to carry to term, however, because in later terminations, the cervix must be dilated much more; this is more likely to weaken the cervix.

Myth #6 *Having a fibroid puts you in a high-risk category for miscarriage.*

Most fibroids do not cause miscarriage. The type

of fibroid that *may* do so is a large one located in or around the endometrial cavity. (This is where implantation occurs in the uterus.) The majority of fibroids are usually insignificant as far as pregnancy is concerned. However, multiple fibroids causing uterine enlargement may be linked with pregnancy loss. Fibroids that cause excessive enlargement of the uterus or abut on the endometrial cavity causing distortion of the cavity may trigger preterm labor, inhibit growth of the placenta, or undergo degeneration, a process where the fibroid breaks down causing inflammation, pain, and often preterm uterine contraction. Fibroid tumors of this size are usually present for many years and women are usually aware of their existence prior to planning a pregnancy. If a woman has a history of fibroids she should consult her gynecologist about their removal prior to a pregnancy. Conversely, a woman who gets regular checkups and is not aware of fibroids in her uterus should not have a problem if a fibroid is diagnosed during pregnancy. Most undiagnosed preexisting fibroids are small and probably insignificant in their relationship to a pregnancy. A woman with one or more small fibroids will be followed during pregnancy with serial sonograms to assess the growth of both the fibroids and the fetus. However, in these cases, a good outcome is usually expected.

Myth #7 Exercising will increase your risk of a miscarriage.

If you have a healthy first-trimester pregnancy and you exercise in a manner to which your body is already accustomed, you won't cause a miscarriage.

However, because physical activity can make the uterus contract, if a pregnancy is unhealthy and is destined to miscarry, the uterine contractions associated with exercise may expel the fetus sooner. This will happen *only* if a miscarriage was already predestined.

Exercise is dangerous only if you do something really strenuous when you are not in good shape. For example, if someone who is fifty pounds overweight and pregnant decides to run five miles to get in shape, that could theoretically be unhealthy for the pregnancy. In that instance oxygen and blood flow could be directed away from the placenta and toward the muscles in the legs, arms, and heart. This disturbance in the placental blood flow may cause a miscarriage. For the average patient who is in good shape and performing moderate activity, exercising is fine. This is not necessarily true in second and third trimesters when activity may have detrimental effects on pregnancy maintenance. There are specific conditions in these trimesters where avoidance of exercise and even bedrest may be required to salvage a pregnancy.

Why then do so many doctors tell women who've miscarried not to exercise during their subsequent pregnancies? Because women who exercise and then miscarry often look back and are convinced that their miscarriage was in some way related to their activity, even though their doctors assure them that it was not. Many doctors will advise women not to exercise so that they won't have to deal with this guilt should a second miscarriage occur.

Myth #8 *Sexual intercourse will cause a miscarriage.*

Intercourse could be problematic in a second or third trimester high-risk pregnancy. However, in a healthy first trimester pregnancy, intercourse is in no way associated with miscarriage. As is the case with exercise, doctors often tell women not to have sex during their first trimester for emotional reasons: It makes women feel as if they're actively doing something to protect their pregnancies and, should something go wrong, they won't be worrying that they miscarried because they had sex the night before the miscarriage happened. But, as with exercise, intercourse will not harm an early healthy pregnancy.

Myth #9 *Taking an airplane trip may cause a miscarriage.*

It has never been scientifically proven that women who fly frequently have any increased risk of miscarriage. This fiction may have arisen from the fact that doctors often tell women not to fly if they have a history of miscarriage, not because flying is dangerous but because the doctors want the women to be nearby just in case they miscarry again and need immediate medical attention.

Myth #10 *Working at a computer all day increases your risk of miscarriage.*

Every so often a number of miscarriages will occur in an office where women work at computers for several hours a day, giving rise to speculation that the computers emit a dangerous type of radiation. Studies have found that daily use of a video terminal does not increase the risks of miscarriage. These outbreaks of miscarriages within a pool of office workers are either random occurrences or may be caused by some environmental or infectious hazards rather than computers.

Myth #11 *Bed rest will help prevent miscarriage.*

Bed rest could delay a miscarriage but it won't prevent one. Most early miscarriages are inevitable.

Now that we've covered the most prevalent myths let's turn to the facts. We'll start with the most basic facts of life, facts with which most of us probably aren't familiar. We all know that pregnancy occurs when a sperm fuses with an egg, but did you know that by the time this penetration is completed, the egg has already undergone two chromosomal divisions, each of these divisions giving rise to an opportunity for a random chromosomal error (the most common cause of miscarriage)? This fact, and other facts of pregnancy, and the physical experience of miscarriage will be explored in the next chapter.

2

▼

PREGNANCY AND MISCARRIAGE

In the belief that you need to understand what has to go right in a pregnancy before you can fully understand what may go wrong, this chapter begins by tracing the steps that must be completed in order for your egg to be fertilized, implant and develop properly.

It then details how your miscarriage may occur should one of those steps not take place correctly.

Finally, it discusses what will be medically recommended if you have one miscarriage, how your next pregnancy will be monitored by your doctor, and what advice will be given should you miscarry again.

HOW A HEALTHY PREGNANCY BEGINS

As a woman, you were born with all the eggs, or primary oocytes, you will ever have, approximately two million of them. Like all the other cells in your body, primary oocytes contain the full number of chromosomes—46. (Chromosomes are microscopic rod-shaped bodies. They carry genes, which convey hereditary characteristics.) Primary oocytes are encased within tiny sacs called *follicles* and lie dormant within your ovaries until, with every menstrual cycle, a few will ripen and mature and one will be released. The process of maturation and release of an egg is called ovulation.

Ovulation

The menstrual cycle is regulated by a series of hormonal events. At the start of each cycle, the *hypothalamus,* a gland in the brain, sends *gonadotrophin-releasing hormone* (GnRH) to the pituitary gland, at the base of the brain. This is the beginning of a hormonal chain reaction. The pituitary then releases another hormone—*follicle-stimulating hormone* (FSH)—which, in turn, signals your ovaries to step up their production of the hormone estrogen.

The increased level of estrogen does two things. First, it causes the endometrium (the lining of the uterus) to thicken, so that it will be able to host a fertilized egg. Second, it causes a few primary oocytes to start ripening in preparation for ovulation. During this ripening process the primary oocytes will undergo (or complete) their first chromosomal division—splitting to form one secondary oocyte and a polar body. The secondary oocyte contains twenty-three chromosomes, the correct number required for fertilization.

After this chromosomal division is completed, your estrogen level rises, and the hypothalamus signals the pituitary to secrete another hormone, known as *luteinizing hormone* (LH). This surge of LH causes one mature follicle to rupture and release the secondary oocyte into the fallopian tube.

This moment is called *ovulation*.

Fertilization

The secondary oocyte will remain alive for twelve to twenty-four hours after ovulation and can be fertilized only during that time. Sperm, however, live longer than eggs. If you had intercourse anywhere up to four days before ovulation, some live sperm may be waiting for the egg within the fallopian tube. Therefore, pregnancy can occur if intercourse happens anytime between four days before ovulation to one day after. (A recent article in the *New England Journal of Medicine* supported the notion that preovulatory intercourse is much more likely to result in conception than postovulatory intercourse, supporting the idea that the egg is maximally viable in its first 12 hours of life.)

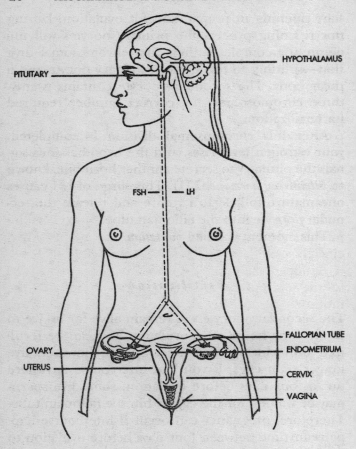

FIGURE 1. The female endocrine and reproductive systems.

At ovulation, the chromosomes in the secondary oocyte begin to divide. If fertilization occurs, the division process is completed to form the mature egg that will fuse with the paternal chromosomes from the sperm.

During the process of fertilization, all of the parental chromosomes pair up with their numerical partners so that "Mom's Chromosome #1" pairs up with "Dad's Chromosome #1"; "Mom's #2" pairs up with "Dad's #2," and so on, all the way down the line to #22. The 23rd pair of chromosomes are the sex chromosomes "X" and/or "Y." Each chromosome is made up of groups of genes, and each gene carries instructions or "codes" for the development of specific characteristics.

Besides contributing half of the genetic material to the pregnancy, the sperm also stimulates the mother's body to create *fetal-blocking antibodies* that protect the pregnancy. Normally, a woman's antibodies attack any substance perceived to be foreign to the system. Fetal-blocking antibodies prevent the mother's other antibodies from recognizing the sperm as foreign and, therefore, rejecting the pregnancy.

The Corpus Luteum

While the chromosomes are pairing up and the fertilized egg is producing fetal-blocking antibodies, an important pregnancy-sustaining structure called the *corpus luteum* is being formed at the site on the ovary where ovulation occurred. The corpus luteum is extraordinarily important since it produces the progesterone needed to sustain the pregnancy at this point. Interestingly, the corpus luteum supports the fertilized egg, and the fertilized egg returns the favor by supporting the corpus luteum via secretion of a hormone called *human chorionic gonadotropin* (HCG). (The presence of HCG is what home pregnancy tests detect and is also what doctors look for in blood tests to confirm pregnancy.)

The progesterone secreted by the corpus luteum serves three very important functions: it prepares the endometrium for implantation, it allows implantation to occur, and it supports the pregnancy for the first eight to ten weeks of gestation, until the placenta becomes fully functional and produces progesterone on its own. (For the purposes of this book, "weeks" is counting from the first day of the last period, not from ovulation. Women tend to think of how far along their pregnancies are in terms of when they ovulated. However, because the presumed date of ovulation can be inaccurate, doctors always count from the first day of the last period, since that date is better known.)

In some women the corpus luteum may be too small to be detected during a physical exam or on a sonogram. When the corpus luteum is large enough to be detected, it is called a *corpus luteum cyst*. This is a normal cyst which will be reabsorbed by the body and will disappear when it is no longer needed.

Implantation

After fertilization, it takes the fertilized egg (also called the *zygote* at this stage) about three days to travel through the fallopian tube to the uterus. Once there, it finds a healthy and hormonally agreeable place along the endometrium and burrows its way in using its outer layer of specialized tissue called *trophoblast*.

This process of embedding in the uterine wall may lead to bleeding due to the disruption of small capillaries in the endometrium. This bleeding is a normal part of the implantation process and may account for the staining that is often seen in the first trimester.

Women may think this staining should occur before the date of their expected period, since that's when implantation is actually occurring. The bleeding *does* occur then, but the blood is often not passed until a few weeks later. The color of blood is often indicative of how old it is: Fresh bleeding is bright red; as the blood ages it turns brown. So, when women see brown staining, that bleeding may have occurred a week or two earlier.

Early Development

Once the zygote has attached itself to the endometrium, the placenta begins to grow. The pregnancy is now referred to as an *embryo*. At four weeks, the cells of the embryo start to differentiate and become specialized. From this point until twelve weeks into the pregnancy, all of the organ systems form. By the end of the first trimester, almost all of the organ systems, except for the brain, are structurally complete although functionally immature. (The brain will continue to grow and alter throughout pregnancy.)

At twelve weeks, the pregnancy is referred to as a *fetus*. After this point, a structural malformation can't occur in any part of the body, except for the brain.

Once your pregnancy has made it to eight weeks, and your embryo has a heartbeat, the risk of miscarriage drops to less than 3 percent. If one miscarries prior to eight weeks little can be done to prevent this first miscarriage, regardless of its cause. Patients with previous miscarriages are evaluated differently, and we will discuss them in Chapter 4.

WHEN SOMETHING GOES WRONG

Although all miscarriages occur because a pregnancy is no longer viable, the way in which the miscarriage occurs can vary symptomatically and in its presentation.

The Three Presentations of Miscarriages

One way a miscarriage may present is as a *missed abortion*. It is called this because, had the woman not been scheduled for a routine sonogram, she would have "missed" the fact that her pregnancy was no longer viable.

If not detected a missed abortion could progress to an *incomplete abortion*. When this happens, the body begins spontaneously expelling the pregnancy but does not expel all of it and, therefore, a dilatation and curettage procedure (D&C) is required to suction out the remaining tissue. Some, but not all, incomplete abortions progress to *complete abortions*. As its name suggests, in this stage of miscarriage the woman's body expels the entire pregnancy, and no medical intervention is necessary. Let's now explore these three stages of miscarriage in detail.

Missed Abortion

Symptoms: Generally typified by a lack of common pregnancy symptoms, e.g., queasiness, tender breasts, and fatigue. Some women may be staining. The pregnancy is no longer viable, but the woman's body has not yet begun to expel it. Any pregnancy complicated by bleeding is termed a *"threatened abortion."* However most threatened abortions result in viable pregnancies.

Many women, however, may experience normal pregnancy symptoms due to elevated HCG levels and yet have a nonviable pregnancy.

Very often the diagnosis is a complete surprise to the mother and doctor.

Diagnosis: If the fetal heartbeat has already been established and then disappears, the woman has definitely miscarried. The fetal heartbeat will never disappear once it's been detected unless the pregnancy has been lost.

Also, any fetus that measures at the proper length for seven weeks of gestation or more but has no heartbeat is definitely not viable. No further evaluation (additional sonograms or blood work) is necessary, but it is often conducted for the patient's peace of mind.

Diagnosing a missed abortion can be more difficult if the miscarriage happens before seven weeks, when a heartbeat is not yet detectable. A woman could mistakenly be told her pregnancy is not viable when it is actually healthy. This could happen if the pregnancy is at an earlier gestational age than the woman thought. For example, a woman may feel certain that she conceived at a particular time based on her last period and her presumed date of ovulation, but, if she ovulated unexpectedly late in that cycle, she could be several days to weeks off on the gestational age she reports to her doctor. This happened to one of my patients who was certain she was eight weeks pregnant at the time of her first visit to my office. Her pregnancy appeared quite abnormal for eight weeks, but could have been normal for six weeks.

In cases like this a repeat sonogram in several days, and/or properly rising serial HCG levels and/or a serum (blood) progesterone level of 15 ng/mL or more can help confirm the health of the pregnancy. (We'll discuss what these levels mean in Chapter 4.)

My patient's HCG level was rising normally, and she turned out to have a healthy six-week pregnancy.

She had simply ovulated two weeks later than she had thought. Thus if your pregnancy doesn't look right for its age but otherwise seems healthy, have your doctor confirm its viability with serial sonograms, serial HCG levels, and/or a progesterone level.

Treatment: If a nonviable pregnancy is six and a half weeks or less and you are staining, your doctor may opt to wait and see if the pregnancy will be expelled spontaneously in the next few days, as it will be in the majority of cases. This is done in the hope of avoiding the slight risks inherent in a D&C.

If, however, you are over six and a half weeks, the pregnancy tissue usually will not be expelled completely on its own. When this happens, the cervix remains open, allowing for the possibility of hemorrhaging and infection. A D&C will lower the risk of complications, and ends the wait for the tissue to pass on its own, thus allowing a woman to begin the grieving process.

Incomplete Abortion

Symptoms: Cramping; the passage of blood and fetal matter; an open cervix. While some tissue has been expelled, some remains inside.

Diagnosis: If the cervix is dilated and bleeding is heavy, the pregnancy is in the process of aborting and cannot be salvaged. If the cervix is not obviously dilated but bleeding is heavy, a sonogram should be performed to confirm that a heartbeat is no longer present or that part of the pregnancy has been passed.

Treatment: A D&C is generally required. As with a

missed abortion, if it's less than six and a half weeks into the pregnancy, the doctor may give you a choice of going home and letting the process complete itself naturally. Generally, this is not recommended since you may not completely pass the tissue on your own, and the longer the dead tissue remains inside when the cervix is open, the higher the risk of hemorrhage and infection. For psychological reasons, many women prefer to have a D&C rather than wait for the miscarriage to complete itself.

Complete Abortion

Symptoms: All the tissue has been passed and the cervix has closed.

Diagnosis: A sonogram is advisable to make sure there's no tissue remaining inside the uterus, because once in a while the cervix will feel as if it is closed when it's not.

Treatment: None. If the pregnancy was known to be intrauterine you will be advised that you will bleed intermittently for a couple of weeks. After a presumed complete abortion, a normal menstrual period should resume in four to six weeks. If it doesn't, it may mean that you've either retained a small amount of pregnancy tissue, which will need to be removed, or that you have an ectopic pregnancy. If a sonogram was never performed to make sure your pregnancy implanted in your uterus, and not in one of your fallopian tubes, your HCG level will be monitored immediately after the miscarriage to make sure it has dropped significantly in a week or two. This is to ensure that what you experienced was actually a miscarriage and not heavy bleeding caused by an ectopic pregnancy.

....

Your Chances of Having a Miscarriage

Each consecutive miscarriage increases your risk of another as follows:

Number of miscarriages	*Your risk is*
0	20 percent
1	24 to 30 percent
2	26 to 40 percent
3	32 to 45 percent
4	40 to 75 percen

....

WHEN DIAGNOSTIC TESTING IS PERFORMED

No matter what type of miscarriage you experienced, your doctor will simply assume that the cause of your first miscarriage was a random, nonrecurring chromosomal abnormality or some other chance event, since these are the causes of most first miscarriages. (These causes are discussed in detail in the following chapter.)

After one miscarriage, most doctors will advise you not to undergo any testing to look for causes of the miscarriage because the workup for habitual abortion (also discussed in detail in the next chapter) is

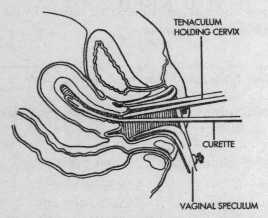

FIGURE 2. *The "C" portion of a postmiscarriage D&C. Prior to inserting a curette—a sharp instrument that looks like a hollow spoon—the doctor has first dilated the cervix with a progression of rods. This opens the cervix to permit access to the uterus. The doctor then suctions out the pregnancy tissue using a clear plastic catheter attached to a suction machine. She uses the curette to scrape the walls of the uterus to make sure there is no remaining tissue.*

expensive. A full workup can cost up to $5,000 and often is not covered by insurance. This workup is usually unwarranted since 80 percent of women who miscarry do not have any underlying physical problems and have subsequent healthy pregnancies. Occasionally, an evaluation of a first miscarriage may be performed if the circumstances surrounding the miscarriage suggest a possible etiology.

Typically, however, you will simply be told to try again after waiting for two to three menstrual cycles so that your uterine lining can rebuild itself.

IF YOU NEED A D&C

A D&C does not require an overnight stay in the hospital. It can be performed either in the doctor's office or in the hospital, depending on the doctor's preference.

You will be told to fast for eight hours before the procedure.

You'll receive intravenous sedation, usually with narcotics and/or anxiety reducing medication (such as Demerol and Valium), and lidocaine may be used locally to anesthetize the cervix. Most women, if they are given the proper amount of medication, sleep during the procedure. If you are awake, you will not remember much afterwards because Valium is an amnesic: It causes you to forget.

The part of the D&C that tends to be uncomfortable is the actual dilatation of the cervix. Again, with good sedation and medication you won't feel much, but, depending on the level of painkillers your doctor uses, you may feel pain similar to bad menstrual cramps.

To dilate the cervix, the doctor uses dilating rods. She will start with one that's just a tiny bit larger in diameter than the endocervical canal opening. She'll place it in the opening, let it sit for a few seconds, then take it out. Then she'll use a slightly larger rod. Each one goes in with a little bit of resistance and sits for a few seconds to stretch the cervix, which will be opened just enough to accommodate a thin plastic catheter attached to a suction machine. The catheter is then inserted into the uterus, and the doctor turns on gentle suction to remove the pregnancy tissue. The catheter tubing is clear so the doctor can see the pregnancy tissue coming out while she does the procedure.

When tissue is no longer being passed through the tube, the doctor will remove the catheter. Then, using a curette—a sharp instrument that looks like a hollow spoon—she will scrape the walls of the uterus to make sure there is no remaining tissue. As she scrapes, the area where the pregnancy was will feel softer than the surrounding walls, which will feel gritty. Once she's gone all the way around your uterus without encountering any retained tissue, she will be done.

The whole procedure, including IV placement and waiting for the medication to take effect, takes about thirty minutes. The doctor's portion of the D&C takes five to ten minutes.

You will be observed for one to four hours to ensure there is no excessive bleeding, unusual pain, or reaction to the analgesics.

You might have some menstrual-type cramping for 24 to 48 hours afterwards and staining or bleeding for up to two weeks, although the bleeding shouldn't be heavy. To lower your risk of infection while your cervix recloses, nothing can be placed in the vagina for two weeks.

Although they occur rarely, a D&C does involve some risks, including:

▼ *Overscraping*, which can lead to scar formation in the uterus known as Asherman's Syndrome
▼ *Perforation* of the uterus by the curette or suction catheter

▼ *Infection* caused by bacteria from the vagina entering the endometrial cavity. While uncommon, this risk can be reduced with the use of prophylactic antibiotics

▼ *Bleeding* from retained tissue.

YOUR SECOND PREGNANCY

If you miscarried your previous pregnancy and are pregnant again, your doctor may want to see you very early, usually at four and a half to five weeks of gestation. This is not because she would necessarily be able to save the pregnancy should something go wrong again, because the only time she might be able to save it is if your problem is a low serum (blood) progesterone level, which can sometimes be supplemented effectively. (See Chapter 4 for more information on progesterone.)

Your doctor will want to schedule an earlier appointment this time to try to diagnose a loss before you begin expelling it so that the tissue can be saved and sent for genetic testing. This type of testing is done by taking live cells from the pregnancy, putting them in culture flasks, and allowing them to grow for several weeks. Individual cells are then extracted, and a chromosomal analysis is performed on them. The sooner the pregnancy tissue is obtained after the loss, the more apt the cells will be to grow in the lab.

ROUTINE TESTING

In your first pregnancy your blood was routinely screened for anemia, infection, blood type to check your Rh factor, hepatitis B, syphilis, rubella, infections that are known to have implications for your pregnancy and/or fetus and for other problems as needed. For instance, if you own a cat or eat undercooked meat, you were probably screened for toxoplasmosis. If you work with young children and, therefore, are often exposed to viruses, you may have been screened for cytomegalovirus. (These infections are covered in detail in Chapter 3.) A sonogram may not have been performed if you were considered to be a low-risk patient.

In this pregnancy, however, the doctor will perform a transvaginal sonogram and bloodwork that may include measurements of your HCG and progesterone levels. If your progesterone level is under 10 ng/mL, your doctor may choose to supplement it immediately.

You will be asked to return to the office in two to four days for a repeat sonogram and another HCG level to make sure your HCG level is rising properly. The level should increase from 1.6 to 2 times its previous level every two days in the early weeks of pregnancy. As a general guideline if it's 1,000 on Monday it should be at least 1,600 on Wednesday. If the HCG level is not rising normally, it could mean that the pregnancy isn't healthy.

ANOTHER MISCARRIAGE

By the sixth week of pregnancy, a fetus should be visible on the sonogram. If the sonographic appearance is abnormal in conjunction with an abnormally rising HCG and an abnormal serum progesterone level, your pregnancy will be found to be nonviable. It's important to remember that in uncertain situations all three—a sonogram, HCG level, and a progesterone level—may be necessary to diagnose a nonviable pregnancy. If your pregnancy is found to be nonviable, you will be diagnosed as having had a missed abortion. A D&C will be performed and you will be asked if you want the pregnancy tissue to be sent for chromosomal analysis.

At this point, since you've suffered two consecutive miscarriages, you may want to consider undergoing what's called a "habitual abortion workup" to see if an underlying problem might be causing you to miscarry.

Until recently, standard medical wisdom was not to send a woman for a workup until she'd suffered three consecutive miscarriages. Only then was the woman determined to be a habitual or recurrent aborter. As discussed in Chapter 1, with so many women conceiving later in life, more and more doctors are sending women for a habitual-abortion workup after two consecutive miscarriages. The order in which your evaluation will be conducted will depend on your personal medical history. So, before you embark on your testing, try to think of any unusual symptoms you may have experienced. For example, unusually light periods following a D&C (which may have been performed after your first miscarriage) and difficulty getting pregnant may indicate Asherman's Syndrome (scarring of the uterus). Make sure to report all symptoms to your doctor. Doing this will lessen the number of tests you'll need to undergo and will give you an answer sooner.

Let us now turn to the causes of miscarriage. In the next chapter, we will cover the causes of random, nonrecurring miscarriages.

3

▼

THE CAUSES OF SPORADIC MISCARRIAGES

If you have had just one miscarriage, the cause will most often be unknown. One can only speculate as to what went wrong with the pregnancy. Sometimes, however, speculation may be accurate and may cause you to take important steps to make sure you do not miscarry again.

If you are like most women, you can assume that the cause of your miscarriage was a chromosomal abnormality, since that is what causes most sporadic miscarriages. However, if you had a high fever early in pregnancy, you may come to believe that an infection caused your miscarriage. In either instance, and also if during the month that you were pregnant your progesterone level was too low, there was no way you could have predicted the event and nothing you could have done to prevent it.

There are other scenarios as well. Your pregnancy may have been unplanned. Therefore, by the time you found out you were pregnant you may not have had sufficient time to stop taking potentially harmful medications. You may have had surgery without knowing you were pregnant, thereby exposing your fetus to potentially harmful anesthetics. Or you may have been exposed to high levels of environmental or occupational toxins.

If pesticides or chemicals are the suspected cause of your miscarriage, it is important for you to do everything you can to make sure you are not exposed to those same substances during your next pregnancy. For instance, if you work in a dry cleaning store, you may want to change jobs before your next pregnancy.

If any of the above-mentioned scenarios apply to you, you may be blaming yourself for your miscarriage. It is important for you to realize that since you were unaware you were pregnant or that your environment was hazardous to your pregnancy, there was nothing you could have done to protect your pregnancy. You are not to blame for your miscarriage.

Miscarriages may also be caused by excessive smoking or by caffeine or alcohol consumption. If you are a heavy smoker or drink large amounts of caffeine or alcohol, or abuse other illicit substances you must decide before your next pregnancy if you are prepared to dramatically reduce or preferably eliminate these behaviors.

FIVE REASONS FOR
MISCARRIAGE

This chapter will help you try to find a reason for your miscarriage. We will explore, in order of their frequency of occurrence, the causes of random miscarriages, including nonrecurring chromosomal abnormalities; infections; cigarettes, caffeine, and alcohol; transient hormonal deficiencies; and environmental hazards such as pesticides, chemicals, anesthetics, and medications. We will discuss each cause in detail, examining its frequency of occurrence and its role in pregnancy loss. Further, where applicable, we will discuss symptoms, diagnosis, and treatment.

Nonrecurring Chromosomal Abnormalities

Fifty to 60 percent of all miscarriages are caused by some type of chromosomal abnormality. When a pregnancy is chromosomally abnormal, its genetic material sends out invalid coding, or instructions, for embryonic growth, thereby making the pregnancy nonviable. In short, the pregnancy simply cannot develop the way its chromosomes are telling it to, and so the pregnancy dies.

Random chromosomal errors cannot be anticipated, treated, or prevented.

Although errors in chromosomal division can occur in either the egg or the sperm, they most commonly arise in the egg. This is because women generally release only one egg each month, and that's the egg that's going to be fertilized, even if there's a chromosomal error in it. Men, on the other hand, produce millions of sperm in the semen, and the healthy sperm tend to reach the egg first.

The random chromosomal error that most frequently causes miscarriage is called *nondisjunction*. This is when the chromosomes in the egg split unevenly either during the egg's first division, around the time of ovulation, or during the second division, when it is being fertilized. These uneven splits result in the following types of errors:

1. *Trisomy:* A fertilized egg with a trisomy will have one chromosome too many somewhere along its lineup of 23 chromosomal pairs. Of all first trimester pregnancies that are found to be chromosomally abnormal, 50 percent are trisomies. The plurality of these are Trisomy 16 and 21, the latter of which results in Down's Syndrome.
2. *Monosomies:* The fertilized egg has only *one* chromosome where there should have been a pair. This results in a total of 45 chromosomes. Twenty percent of all first trimester chromosomal abnormalities are monosomies.

   All monosomies, except for those involving the X chromosome, are lethal to the pregnancy and the fetus will always abort in the first trimester. Occasionally, however, female fetuses with only one X chromosome (XO instead of XX) will survive to term and be born with Turner's Syndrome. Girls born with Turner's Syndrome have a group of associated abnormalities: Their chests are wide and flat, they never develop sexually, and they are infertile. They may also be mentally retarded.

There are other types of chromosomal errors as well. These include the following:

1. *Triploidy:* The fertilized egg has a chromosomal count of 69. It is generally believed that this error results when two sperm fertilize an egg. Twenty percent of all first trimester chromosomal abnormalities are due to triploidy.
2. *Tetraploidy and all others:* In tetraploidy, the fertilized egg has 92 chromosomes. This means that either three sperm fertilized the egg, or improper cleavage of the zygote occurred. Other, less frequent chromosomal errors can occur, but they are rare and too numerous to mention here.

Why Chromosomal Errors Increase as a Woman Ages

Sporadic chromosomal errors can happen to any woman of any age, but they rise dramatically after a woman reaches age 35. This is because your eggs have been in your ovaries since you were born, so if you don't have a child before you're 35, all of your eggs are 35 years old. The older the egg, the more of a tendency it has to make chromosomal errors when it divides.

The vast majority of random chromosomal errors miscarry before the eighth week. Only certain trisomies and abnormalities of the sex chromosomes generally make it to term. For example, 20 percent of Down's Syndrome and 4 to 5 percent of Turner's Syndrome, respectively.

As explained in the previous chapter, since chromosomal abnormalities are so common, if this is your first miscarriage doctors will often simply assume that the cause of the miscarriage was a random chromosomal error. A true diagnosis—arrived at from testing the fetal tissue for genetic defects—will almost never be sought. After your second consecutive miscarriage, if the tissue is salvageable, it will usually be sent for chromosomal analysis.

There is no treatment for this type of miscarriage. You will simply be told to try again. Assuming there is no other underlying problem, you should have a success rate on your subsequent pregnancy equal to that of the general population.

Infections

The subject of infections and their relationship to miscarriage is a complex one because it is often difficult to assess the connection between a recent infection and the loss of a pregnancy. For example, let's say a woman is six-and-a-half weeks pregnant and develops flulike symptoms. She takes an acetaminophen product such as Tylenol, but her fever still rises over 100.4 degrees, the point at which a fever is believed to be harmful to a pregnancy.

At her next appointment, the fetus is no longer viable. The woman will feel sure that her miscarriage was related to her illness. But there is no way to be certain of that. She may have been one of the 20 percent of women who would have spontaneously miscarried anyway. On the other hand, she may be right—the fever may have injured the pregnancy. Often doctors just don't know.

There are at least six infections, however, that are known to cause malformations in the fetus and increased miscarriage rates *if they are newly acquired during the pregnancy*. These are toxoplasmosis, rubella, cytomegalovirus, an initial infection of herpes, syphilis, and chicken pox.

There are also infections such as parvovirus and mumps that are thought to play a role in miscarriage but that do not cause malformations. In these cases, the infectious agent itself or the fever it causes may have a toxic effect on the fetus.

For all of these infections, statistics as to their frequency of occurrence and their miscarriage rates are not available. If they do cause a miscarriage, the miscarriage tends to happen during the first trimester or early in the second.

Infections that cause malformations in the fetus

Again, it is important to stress that these six infections will cause fetal malformations and, therefore, increased miscarriage rates, *only if they are newly ac-*

quired during the pregnancy. Five of these infections—
toxoplasmosis, rubella, cytomegalovirus, herpes, and
chicken pox—are viruses. Like all viruses, these will
be diagnosed by screening your blood for antibodies
to the viral infection.

Your doctor will check for two types of antibodies:

1. *IgG:* This is an immunoglobulin, a protein made
   in response to an infection. If you've been infected, some level of this antibody will be present
   throughout your lifetime.
2. *IgM:* This is also an immunoglobulin, but it will be
   present only during the acute phase of an illness.
   It is usually not maintained by the body for a long
   time.

The absence of these antibodies reveals that you
have not had the particular infection, and that you
are susceptible to it.

The presence of IgG alone indicates an old infection, or immunity and poses no current risk to the
pregnancy. If you're immune, your fetus is not at risk.

The presence of IgG and IgM together or IgM
alone is more of a concern and may indicate a newly
acquired infection that could cause the pregnancy to
develop abnormally. Since most women in this situation terminate their pregnancies, we do not know
the exact incidence of these anomalies and the associated miscarriage rate.

Toxoplasmosis Toxoplasmosis is caused by a parasite present in infected cat feces and in undercooked

meat. Anyone who owns a cat or eats undercooked meat should be screened for this parasite.

You contract toxoplasmosis via your gastrointestinal tract by touching infected cat litter and then bringing your hands to your mouth or by touching your food with your hands. You can also get it by eating undercooked meat. There are usually no symptoms, although some people have a slight fever, diarrhea, lethargy, and swollen glands. To diagnose toxoplasmosis your blood will be screened for toxoplasma antibodies. If you are pregnant, and have a newly acquired infection, consultation with a specialist regarding treatment options or termination is advised. A previous infection of toxoplasmosis will give you immunity.

Note: If your titer (the name of the measuring unit used when testing for viruses) was negative, you should not change the cat litter during your entire pregnancy; you should keep a distance from the cat; and you should wash your hands after any contact with either the litterbox or the cat. You especially shouldn't let the cat lick you. You should also cook your meat medium or well done. Fetuses exposed to toxoplasma can have many anomalies including growth retardation, microcepaly, mental retardation and blindness.

Rubella This virus is also known as "German measles." A rubella screening is routinely done on all women who are planning to become pregnant or who are newly pregnant. The virus is transmitted through the air when an infected person coughs or sneezes. Since children are now vaccinated against rubella, it is not as common as it was in the past. If you have had rubella, you are immune to it.

Symptoms of rubella are flulike. Diagnosis is made by a blood test for antibody titers. There is no treatment. The illness simply runs its course. The congenital rubella syndrome is characterized by congenital catarracts, heart disease, and mental retardation.

Cytomegalovirus Cytomegalovirus is a flulike virus that is common in children. You should be screened for it if you work closely with children. You catch the illness through bodily secretions by way of your gastrointestinal or respiratory tracts. The symptoms are similar to those of flu. Diagnosis is made by a blood test for antibody titers. There is no treatment. Cytomegalovirus can be reactivated, but this is rare. Only the initial infection is harmful to the pregnancy.

If you're a schoolteacher, day-care worker, or pediatrician, and your antibody titer is negative, try to avoid having close contact with sick kids. If you're a mother and your child develops a fever or a flulike illness, you should try to avoid close physical contact until your child's fever passes. Cytomegalovirus can lead to growth restriction and mental retardation.

Herpes Herpes is a virus that is classified as either Type 1 (most commonly seen in oral infections) or Type 2 (most commonly seen in genital infections). You can catch either type in either bodily location, and both types of primary infections can hurt your pregnancy. As far as we know, recurrent herpes has no bearing on pregnancy except possibly at the time of delivery when a genital lesion could come in contact with the baby as it passes through the birth canal, thus transmitting the infection to the newborn. Anyone who shows symptoms of herpes during their pregnancy should be screened.

Herpes is contracted through skin-to-skin contact with someone who has herpetic lesions. The main symptom will be lesions that look like small, water-filled blisters. With a primary infection you may also feel as if you have the flu. Diagnosis can be suggested by a blood test for antibody titer or confirmed by a positive culture from the lesion. There is no treatment for herpes. Certain medications will lessen the severity and duration of your symptoms, but these medications are not known to be safe to take during pregnancy. Neonatal herpes is associated with a 50 percent mortality rate and significant neurologic disease in the surviving infants.

Syphilis Unlike the other infections known to cause congenital anomalies, syphilis is a virus caused by a microorganism known as a *spirochete* and is transmitted though sexual contact. In the primary stage, you develop a painless lesion known as a *chancre* (a large ulcerative lesion) usually on your genitals. If this stage goes undiagnosed, you may progress to secondary syphilis, which is characterized by a rash most commonly seen on the palms of the hands and soles of the feet. After this, a latent phase may last anywhere from weeks to years. Some people will go on to develop tertiary syphilis, which can cause permanent neurologic and cardiac damage.

All women receiving prenatal care in this country are routinely screened via a blood test for syphilis on their first visit.

Treatment involves one or more injections of Benzathine penicillin, depending on the stage of the disease. With prompt treatment, the chance of successfully curing the disease is excellent. Erythromycin can be substituted for the penicillin-allergic patient. Congenital syphilis is a well-described entity consisting of abnormal dentition, saddle nose, abnormal facies, shin and eye lesions, and mental retardation.

Chicken pox   Chicken pox is a herpes-type virus called *varicella*. It is acquired through contact with respiratory secretions from an infected person, usually a child. Small, itchy blisters spread over the whole body and a fever will develop. You may also have flulike upper respiratory symptoms.

A diagnosis is usually made by the rash and symptoms, but it can be confirmed with a blood test for antibody titers. At the moment, there is no treatment for chicken pox. Now that a vaccine for chicken pox is available, this will probably become less of an issue for pregnant women. Chicken pox can be reactivated in the form of shingles (or herpes zoster), but this reactivation will not harm the fetus. However, an initial first trimester infection of chicken pox can lead to microcephaly, limb-reduction defects, skin lesions, and mental retardation.

Next, we will discuss several infectious illnesses thought to play a role in miscarriage, but whose role is less certain.

Mumps

Mumps is a viral infection of the salivary glands that causes abnormalities in the placenta, but it's not known how or why. These abnormalities are what may cause a miscarriage. Once you've had mumps you become immune.

You can catch this virus through contact with saliva or respiratory secretions from an infected person. Flulike symptoms will appear, as will swollen lymph nodes mostly in the neck. Diagnoses is made by a blood test for antibody titers and symptoms, and there is no treatment.

The miscarriage rate is 40 percent. Those patients whose pregnancies continue after an acute mumps infection are not thought to be at any further risk for pregnancy complications.

Parvovirus

Parvovirus is also called the "Fifth Disease." It's more prevalent in the spring and winter. After having it once, you become immune. You contract parvovirus from the saliva or respiratory secretions of an infected person. You will have an intensely flushed face on the first day. On the second and third day a rash will appear first on the legs and arms and then on the rest of the body. Diagnosis will be made based on symptoms and then confirmed with a blood test for antibody titers. There is no treatment.

There is a high rate of miscarriage during the acute phase of the illness. If your pregnancy continues, serious complications to the fetus may develop later in the pregnancy, and you will be followed with serial sonograms to assess the condition of the fetus.

Listeria

Listeria is a bacterial infection acquired by eating contaminated foods, especially meat or unpasteurized dairy products. Usually there are no symptoms, but you may feel as though you have the flu, with fever and back or muscle aches. Clinically, this bacteria is difficult to distinguish from other bacteria. If you've recently eaten unpasteurized cheese, have a fever and flulike symptoms, a blood test will be done to see if the bacteria grows in the lab. Treatment consists of medications in the penicillin family. Your pregnancy should be fine if you receive prompt treatment. Listeria is one of the few infections known to cross the placenta and may lead to fetal infection and amnionitis.

Lyme Disease

Lyme disease is caused by a spirochete similar to the organism that causes syphilis. It is contracted by being bitten by an infected deer tick. Initially, a distinct circular rash will appear, usually on the limbs. If untreated this may be followed weeks later by meningitis, migrating joint pain or Bell's facial palsy, which, if not treated, may be followed months or years later by neurologic, cardiac, or arthritic manifestations. If a blood test is positive you will be treated with a form of penicillin. The usual treatment is with tetracycline but this is not safe to take during pregnancy.

Because this is a relatively newly identified illness (first described in 1977), knowledge of its effect on pregnancies is limited. It is believed to cause malformations in the fetus, and, therefore, prompt treatment is essential. Doctors don't have any concrete advice to give to women who become infected with Lyme disease during pregnancy. You may be referred to an infectious disease specialist, and your pregnancy will be followed with repeat sonograms.

Other infections

Under this category fall all infections that are associated with high fever, including the flu, because the high fever is thought to be dangerous for the pregnancy. Basically, any organism that can cause fever can cause miscarriage. Anyone who has a high or sustained (over 100.4 F.) fever during pregnancy should try to control the fever with an acetaminophen analgesic such as Tylenol® and contact their doctor to discuss symptoms and possible evaluation.

If you get flulike symptoms and a high fever during pregnancy, you may want to establish that you don't have any of the known worrisome viruses because of their potential to cause congenital anomalies. If your infection is not known to be harmful to pregnancy, your fever has passed, and your pregnancy has progressed, you can assume that your pregnancy was not harmed by the fever.

Cigarettes, Caffeine, and Alcohol

Cigarettes, caffeine, and alcohol have all been shown to increase your risk of miscarriage incrementally, depending on how much you consume.

As a general guideline, cigarette smoking will increase your risk of miscarriage approximately 1.2 times for every ten cigarettes smoked per day. Your risk of miscarriage due to caffeine intake will increase 1.017 times for every cup of coffee consumed per day. Alcohol will increase your risk by 1.26 per drink per day.

The studies all reach the same basic conclusion—the more you smoke, drink alcohol, or consume caffeine the more your risk of miscarriage increases. So what does this mean for you? An occasional cigarette, glass of wine, or cup of coffee or glass of caffeinated soda won't cause you to miscarry, but continued heavy usage very well might.

With cigarettes, it's believed that the carbon monoxide in the cigarette smoke has a direct toxic effect on the fetus. Carbon monoxide binds to blood preferentially over oxygen, so your blood chooses the carbon monoxide in the cigarette smoke over the oxygen in the air. Your blood will not be carrying enough oxygen to the fetus, and, therefore, the fetus will die.

Alcohol is believed to raise the instances of miscarriage either because it is toxic to the fetus or because it causes malformations in the developing brain. It is generally advised that pregnant women not drink in the first trimester and limit intake to less than one drink per week in the second and third trimesters.

And, finally, caffeine. New studies on the effects of caffeine are published frequently, and while one study will say you can drink as much as you want and it will have no bearing on pregnancy, another will say that a cup of coffee a day will cause a miscarriage. On the whole, you'll be safe cutting your use down to 2 cups or less per day.

Transient Hormonal Deficiencies

Transient means not permanent. Many women will have transient hormonal deficiencies during some of their menstrual cycles. This means that during those cycles they are not producing enough progesterone to properly prepare their endometrium for the implantation of the fertilized egg. If they happen to get pregnant during that cycle, they will lose the pregnancy. Transient hormonal deficiencies are impossible to diagnose since they may not be repeated for many more cycles.

If your doctor suspects that a low level of progesterone has caused your miscarriage, she may put you on progesterone supplements the next time you are pregnant. Doing so is controversial and will be discussed in detail in the next chapter. If a woman's hormonal deficiencies are permanent, as opposed to transient, they will cause her to repeatedly miscarry. This will also be discussed in the next chapter.

Environmental Hazards

The reasons behind other random, nonrecurring miscarriages tend to be such things as soaking for an extended period in a hot tub (which can raise your core temperature in a way similar to a fever) or something in your environment. The following "environmental" hazards are almost always avoidable.

Pesticides/chemicals/lead

Many, if not all, of the toxic pesticides or chemicals in our environment are thought to be potentially detrimental to pregnancy. Our exposure to these pesticides or chemicals is often for short periods of time, or in minimal concentrations, and therefore is not likely to adversely affect the fetus. However, if you are aware of toxic substances in your work or home environment, minimize skin contact and respiratory inhalation as much as possible. Consult your physician about each substance's specific toxicity.

As for lead, toxic blood levels of this tasteless, odorless metal have definitely been linked to miscarriage. You are at risk for lead poisoning if the pipes for your drinking water are made of lead or if your dwelling or place of work was built before 1978, when lead paint was taken off the market. The latter risk exists only if the paint is chipping or cracking. In those instances, you may be breathing in paint dust contaminated with lead. There is no treatment for lead poisoning. To protect yourself and your family you'll have to decontaminate your living or working environment.

THE CAUSES OF SPORADIC MISCARRIAGES   61

Ideally, your lead levels should be screened pre-conceptually. If your lead levels are high you should wait for them to return to normal before becoming pregnant. If you are already pregnant and are found to have high levels of lead in your blood, remove yourself from the lead-infested environment until it has been decontaminated. Change your drinking pipes (or drink only bottled water) and hire only certified professionals to remove your lead paint.

If you have lead poisoning and do not miscarry, and eliminate any future exposure to lead, your pregnancy should continue uneventfully.

Anesthetics

If possible, put off any medical or dental procedure requiring general anesthesia. If the procedure can't be avoided, local anesthesia is fine as a rule, but general anesthesia should wait until you've passed your first trimester. It's not known why anesthesia can increase your miscarriage rate, but it is not associated with fetal anomalies. If you do have to undergo a procedure and your pregnancy continues, you don't have to worry about the pregnancy.

Medications

There are numerous medications to avoid during pregnancy. Any and all medications that you take regularly should be discussed with your physician prior to conception.

For peace of mind, remember that all of the causes discussed in this chapter—except for those that are within your power to either control or remove yourself from—are unlikely to be repeated. If your miscarriage was caused by a random event, your chances of carrying your next pregnancy to term are excellent.

If, however, you have consecutively miscarried two or more pregnancies, your miscarriages are most likely not random events. You may have an underlying physical condition that, until treated, will cause you to miscarry again and again. We will examine these conditions in the next chapter.

4

▼

THE CAUSES OF RECURRING MISCARRIAGES

About 20 percent of women who miscarry will do so repeatedly. A woman traditionally became classified as a recurring or habitual aborter after three consecutive miscarriages. These days, with so many women becoming pregnant later in life and, therefore, having less time in which to bear children, more and more doctors are classifying women as habitual aborters after two miscarriages. Once you are classified a habitual aborter, you will then be sent for diagnostic testing.

The unfortunate news about recurring miscarriages is that women will often have to suffer at least two miscarriages before any diagnostic testing will be performed to try to unearth the underlying physical condition.

The good news is that 75 percent of the time, a cause for these miscarriages can be found, almost all of the causes are treatable, and their treatments have up to an 80 percent success rate.

The well-established causes of repeat miscarriages are:
▼ hormonal imbalances
▼ anatomic defects in a woman's reproductive system
▼ infectious organisms
▼ chromosomal abnormalities carried by one or both parents that are repeatedly passed along to their fetuses
▼ antiphospholipid syndrome

This chapter will explain each condition in detail, including its miscarriage rate, when the miscarriage would happen, how a diagnosis is made, treatment, and the success rate of that treatment.

HORMONAL IMBALANCE

Hormonal or endocrine imbalances, caused either by luteal phase defect, thyroid disease or diabetes, account for about 30 percent of recurrent miscarriages.

Luteal Phase Defect (LPD)

LPD accounts for about 25 percent of all recurrent miscarriages. A woman with this condition does not produce enough progesterone after ovulation to properly prepare her endometrial lining to accept a fertilized egg for implantation. Sometimes women who believe they are infertile are actually conceiving but, due to a luteal phase defect, are miscarrying their pregnancies at a very early stage, before they even know they are pregnant.

If the defect is severe, the miscarriage will happen before, or around the time of, the expected period. If it's mild, the miscarriage may not happen for six to eight weeks. LPD won't cause a miscarriage after 8–10 weeks because the placenta is producing progesterone by that time, and the mother's ovarian progesterone is no longer necessary to support the pregnancy.

Diagnosing LPD

To properly diagnose LPD your doctor must perform two consecutive endometrial biopsies. This is because many normal women will have an occasional LPD. For some reason, they may have a low progesterone level during a particular cycle, but that low progesterone level is not indicative of what their bodies do all the time. Two consecutively diagnosed LPDs, on two consecutive cycles however, could indicate a recurring problem.

The endometrial biopsy will be done in your doctor's office two to three days before your anticipated period. There is no dilatation of the cervix, and no anesthetic is used. A tiny plastic catheter with a plunger at the end will be inserted into the uterus. The plunger will create suction, and the doctor will twirl the catheter in her fingers while moving it up and down the uterine cavity until the full length of the catheter is filled with endometrial tissue. You will feel some moderate menstrual-type cramping. The procedure takes two minutes.

Your endometrial tissue will be sent to a pathologist who will then date the tissue. This means that, based primarily on the appearance of your blood vessels and endometrial tissue, he will tell you what day of your menstrual cycle you should be in. More than a two-day lag is considered abnormal. For example, if you have a 28-day cycle and your endometrium was biopsied on day 25, but the lab results said your endometrium looked like day 19, your doctor will conclude that you are not producing enough progesterone to prepare the lining of the uterus for implantation.

For accurate dating of the endometrium, it is imperative that you call your doctor and tell her when your next period actually begins. While the pathologist will have dated your endometrium based on your previous cycle, the dating is actually much more accurate if you count backwards from the day your next period begins. That first day of bleeding will be referred to as day 28, and your doctor will count backwards to when your biopsy was performed. This dating is much more accurate because when the specimen was taken the doctor could only presume your date of ovulation based on your previous cycle. While ovulation can be irregular, your period will always begin 14 to 16 days after ovulation. You may have ovulated late during the cycle in which the biopsy was done, and that would have thrown off the pathologist's dating.

Note: You may be advised to abstain from intercourse for psychological reasons during the menstrual cycles in which the endometrial biopsies are performed. If you are pregnant while the procedure is done, there's a very remote chance that during the biopsy the implantation site could be disrupted. By abstaining, you won't be worrying that you conceived and that the procedure disrupted the pregnancy.

Luteal phase defect can be treated in one of two ways, either with clomiphene citrate or with progesterone supplements.

Treating LPD with Clomiphene Citrate

Clomiphene citrate (brand name Clomid or Serophene) is the preferred treatment. It's taken orally on days five through nine of the menstrual cycle. You take it each cycle until you get pregnant. Most women take it for 3 to 6 months, since this is considered the normal amount of time required to conceive. Once you get pregnant, no further treatment will be necessary.

Clomiphene citrate works at the level of the hypothalamus to interfere with estrogen detection. This causes the body to think it's in a lower estrogen state than it really is at the beginning of the menstrual cycle, causing the pituitary to produce more follicle stimulating hormone (FSH), which will then cause the ovary to produce more estrogen and recruit more follicles. Estrogen and progesterone production are interlinked. Because you'll have an increase of estrogen and follicle production in the first half of the cycle, you will have increased progesterone production in the second half of the cycle. This increased progesterone production will lead to proper development of the endometrial lining and, therefore, allow implantation to occur.

Clomiphene citrate is the preferred treatment because you don't have to worry about the timing of the treatment in terms of when ovulation occurs. Again, it's always given on days five through nine of the cycle, regardless of when ovulation occurs, and it will not delay the onset of the next period, which progesterone treatment may do. (A discussion of this method of treatment follows.)

Bad PMS symptoms are common side effects when using clomiphene citrate. They include breast tenderness, fluid retention, and irritability.

Clomiphene citrate has been in use since 1960, but its possible long-term effects on the women taking it and/or on their children aren't fully known.

Your chance of having twins rises to 10 to 12 percent since the increased estrogen production caused by clomiphene citrate will often cause more than one egg to mature and be released during ovulation. It is not clear whether it may increase your risk of ovarian cancer, and this is still under investigation. It has not been linked to any malformation or known problems in the children of women who have taken the drug.

In a tiny percentage of women, clomiphene citrate will have an adverse effect on cervical mucus. Those women who have mucus problems that may affect their ability to conceive (their mucus is either too dry or deficient in quantity) may exacerbate their problem by taking this drug.

Indeed, if you're taking clomiphene citrate and have difficulty conceiving, your doctor may want to do a postcoital test during one of the first two cycles that you're on the drug, just to make sure that your mucus is healthy. To ensure accurate results, your spouse should first undergo a semen analysis to confirm that his sperm is inherently healthy.

To do the postcoital test your doctor will tell you to have intercourse on the day before, or the day of, ovulation. These are days during which your cervical mucus should be most abundant and receptive to sperm. You will then see your doctor between three and twelve hours after intercourse. She will take a small amount of mucus out of your cervical canal and look at it under a microscope to check if the sperm are healthy and swimming in a forward direction. A cervical mucus problem would be diagnosed if the sperm were dead, shaking in place, swimming in circles, or absent, since thick, unreceptive mucus can kill sperm or prevent normal motility.

Treating LPD with Progesterone

Progesterone supplements are most often delivered by vaginal suppositories, but sometimes they are given by injection or by oral micronized progesterone. Although clomiphene citrate is the easiest and usually preferred way of treating LPD, some doctors prescribe progesterone.

If your doctor prescribes progesterone for a diagnosed LPD, keep in mind that ideally the supplements should be begun a day or two after ovulation. If you supplement progesterone too close to ovulation or you hit the day of ovulation, the progesterone may interfere with fertilization or the early process of the pregnancy. (This is why most doctors prefer clomiphene citrate.) You want to make sure fertilization is over and done with before you start the progesterone. Also, if the supplements are begun at the time of the missed period (i.e., the moment you realize you're pregnant, which is when some doctors incorrectly tell you to begin taking them), it may be too late to correct the problem caused by LPD.

You will need to supplement your progesterone through approximately the eighth to tenth week after the start of your last menstrual period, beginning approximately 48 hours after ovulation. You will need to use an ovulation predictor kit to time this properly. Once you are past the tenth week after the start of your last menstrual period, the placenta will be fully functional and producing the progesterone needed to sustain the pregnancy.

Premenstrual-type bloating and fluid retention are the most common side effects. Also, your period may be delayed. This can be stressful because you may incorrectly think you are pregnant.

Progesterone supplements will also often delay a miscarriage that's destined to happen. Nonviable pregnancies will cause you to have a low progesterone level, which will cause the body to begin miscarrying. By raising the progesterone levels with supplements, the body will not be getting the proper signals from the nonviable pregnancy and, therefore, will not expel the pregnancy promptly.

Note: Because progesterone supplementation must be taken a day or two after ovulation, a woman with an irregular cycle will have a difficult time with progesterone and will have to use an ovulation predictor kit for extended periods. In this case, clomiphene citrate is definitely preferable.

Pure progesterone doesn't carry any risks as far as we know. Chemical or synthetic progestins on the other hand may have other chemicals in the base of the product that may not be safe for the pregnancy or may negatively affect the fetus.

The Uncertainty Surrounding Progesterone

Sometimes after women miscarry, their doctors tell them to come in as soon as they know they're pregnant again so that they can be started on progesterone suppositories. These doctors figure that since all women have low levels of progesterone during some of their cycles, and that since pure progesterone is a natural substance that can't hurt either the woman or the pregnancy, it couldn't hurt to supplement the progesterone in this manner. Although this sounds harmless, doing this is actually quite controversial.

The first and most important thing for you to know is that if you have a luteal phase defect, supplementing your progesterone at the time of your missed period is the wrong way to treat it. To properly treat a luteal phase defect, progesterone must be supplemented approximately two days after ovulation. If you supplement it at the time of the missed period, your pregnancy may already have begun to be lost.

If you have *not* been diagnosed as having luteal phase defect but are pregnant and have low levels of progesterone in your blood, it is debatable whether or not your progesterone should be supplemented.

Most doctors, if they document a low level of progesterone in pregnant women who do not have diagnosed LPD, will give them supplements because it's hard not to. Put yourself in the doctor's shoes: A patient has come into the office and is spotting and cramping but, sonographically, the pregnancy looks healthy. The only thing wrong is that the level of progesterone in the patient's blood is too low. What would you do?

Most doctors would feel obligated to treat that low level of progesterone because so many things are still unknown about how a pregnancy is maintained. It's possible that the corpus luteum could function well for a while, producing enough progesterone to support a very early pregnancy and then degenerate prematurely producing inadequate levels of progesterone for further development.

In some studies, supplementing low progesterone levels at this point in a pregnancy seems to work. But it has never been definitely documented that it was the progesterone that saved the pregnancy. Something else may have been wrong with the pregnancy that corrected itself, and the fact that the woman was given progesterone may have been coincidental.

If pure progesterone is a natural substance and using it can't hurt your pregnancy, why wouldn't all doctors prescribe it for you if your progesterone level is low? Because low progesterone levels are often a sign of pregnancies that are unhealthy for reasons that have nothing to do with progesterone.

For example, if you have a chromosomally abnormal fetus that's not growing properly, you'll have low progesterone production simply because the pregnancy is not healthy. Supplementing that low progesterone level wouldn't make sense, because you're not going to correct a chromosomal defect by raising the level of progesterone. Raising that level may cause you to carry an unhealthy pregnancy longer and would delay the onset of an inevitable miscarriage. (This would be frustrating and emotionally painful.)

What should you do if your pregnancy seems to be in trouble, your progesterone level is documented to be low, but you don't have a diagnosed luteal phase defect? Speak to your doctor about the risks and benefits of supplementing your progesterone. That decision has to be made on an individual basis.

It is important to stress again, however, that if you *do* have a diagnosed luteal phase defect, you can't wait until you miss your period to start the progesterone. With a known luteal phase defect, progesterone supplementation must begin several days after ovulation in order for implantation to occur properly.

Thyroid Disease

Your thyroid is a gland that works like a thermostat, producing two basic thyroid hormones, the most important of which is thyroxine. Located at the base of the neck, the thyroid regulates your metabolism (how you burn calories for energy). The secretion of thyroid hormones is controlled by the pituitary and the portion of the brain above the pituitary called the hypothalamus. If you remember our discussion in Chapter 2, the hypothalamus and the pituitary are also responsible for secreting the hormones that regulate the menstrual cycle, ovulation, and pregnancy. It is believed that significant derangements in thyroid function will affect the production of these pregnancy hormones, which in turn will affect your ability to maintain your pregnancy or, in some cases, even to conceive.

There are two types of thyroid disease: *hypothyroidism*, in which your thyroid doesn't produce enough thyroid hormone, and *hyperthyroidism*, in which it produces too much. Only hypothyroidism has been clearly linked to spontaneous abortion. While some researchers think that hyperthyroidism may also be a cause of spontaneous abortion, this has not been clearly established.

The reason hypothyroidism causes spontaneous abortion is unclear, but the most generally accepted theory is as follows: If you're producing low levels of thyroid hormone, you're going to produce very large amounts of thyroid stimulating hormone. When your thyroid stimulating hormone is greatly increased, it may interfere with the pituitary gland's production of follicle-stimulating hormone. With FSH diminished, your ovary will not function as well. Because your ovary won't be functioning properly, you won't be creating enough estrogen, or enough follicles. Without enough estrogen, you won't create a healthy corpus luteum, which, in turn, means you won't create enough progesterone for implantation to occur properly.

Thyroid disease is often an immune system malfunction. Basically, the immune system fails to recognize the thyroid gland as part of the body and sends antibodies to attack it. The disease accounts for about 5 percent or less of recurrent miscarriages. The miscarriage would generally happen prior to the tenth week of pregnancy. The presence of antithyroid antibodies is a marker for spontaneous abortion. Hypothyroidism without antibodies is probably not associated with miscarriage.

Symptoms of thyroid disease

The symptoms of thyroid disease are often overlooked or misdiagnosed since they so often mimic the symptoms of other illnesses or of too much stress in your life. Remember that certain types of thyroid disease are familial so if you have thyroid disease in your family you should be especially on the lookout for the symptoms.

Hypothyroidism causes your whole body to slow down because too little thyroid hormone is produced. Its symptoms are fatigue, weight gain, constipation, poor concentration, feeling cold all the time, dry skin and hair, and depression. You may also have longer menstrual periods with a heavier flow. You may have difficulty conceiving and maintaining a pregnancy.

Hyperthyroidism causes your body to function in high gear because too much thyroid hormone is produced. Symptoms of hyperthyroidism include difficulty sleeping, weight loss, anxiety, irritability, a racing heartbeat, more frequent bowel movements, and feeling warm. Your menstrual periods may be shorter than usual with a lighter flow.

In both types of thyroid disease, your thyroid may feel enlarged.

Diagnosing thyroid disease

A blood test to measure the level of thyroid stimulating hormone (TSH) secreted by the pituitary gland is used to check for thyroid disease. When the thyroid is underactive, TSH levels will be high; when it's overactive TSH levels will be low.

Treating thyroid disease

You should be referred to an endocrinologist (a specialist in diseases of the glands) for treatment.

For hypothyroidism you would take thyroid replacement hormone in the form of thyroxine. This usually means taking one pill every day for the rest of your life. If you were on this therapy before pregnancy, your dosage of the drug may now need to be adjusted because of the normal hormonal changes that pregnancy brings.

For hyperthyroidism, the thyroid itself has to be

treated. Methods of treatment depend on the extent of the disease and whether or not you are pregnant at the time of diagnosis. Most women are treated with radioactive iodine (in capsule or liquid form), which damages overproductive thyroid cells, causing a decrease in hormone levels.

The low doses of radioactivity are safe *except* during pregnancy. If you require radioactive iodine, you should not conceive for six months after the conclusion of treatment. If you are pregnant, your endocrinologist may recommend other drugs to turn off excess hormone production or surgery to remove the thyroid, followed by hormone replacement.

The success depends on when you're diagnosed and how early in the pregnancy your problem was corrected. If it was corrected before you conceived, you'll have the same miscarriage rate as the general population.

A small percentage of women have been found to have antithyroid antibodies in the absence of thyroid disease. These antibodies are linked to an increased risk of miscarriage although the mechanism of action is unclear. No treatment is available at present.

Diabetes

Diabetes arises when the pancreas is unable to produce enough insulin to control glucose levels in your blood. It is sometimes a cause of miscarriage, but its real danger lies in fetal anomalies. Diabetes will cause a miscarriage only if it's late-stage or very poorly controlled. Women with late-stage diabetes are usually advised not to get pregnant.

One in 200 pregnant women will have preexisting diabetes. Those women who develop diabetes *during* their pregnancies (known as gestational diabetes) do not have an increased risk of miscarriage or malformations.

Diagnosing diabetes

Diabetes is diagnosed with a glucose tolerance test. After an overnight fast of 8-12 hours a fasting blood sugar level is drawn. One then ingests a 100 gram glucose load and three hourly sugar levels are drawn. Two or more abnormal values are consistent with a diagnosis of diabetes. Often a one hour 50 gram glucose level is used as a pre-screening test to see who requires the three-hour GTT (glucose tolerance test).

Treating diabetes

Treatment of the condition includes dietary restriction of refined sugars and carbohydrates and may include oral or injectable insulin, depending on the severity of the illness. However oral medications are not used during pregnancy.

For the patient with diabetes in good control, and who lacks organ damage (i.e., compromise of kidney or heart function or vascular disease) secondary to the diabetes, the miscarriage rates are the same as for the general population. Yet, even with good preconception sugar control, women with preexisting diabetes still have a two-fold increased risk of fetal malformations.

ANATOMIC DEFECTS

Under this category falls everything that can be *structurally* wrong with a woman's reproductive system that would cause miscarriage: uterine anomalies, Asherman's syndrome, and an incompetent cervix.

Uterine Anomalies

When you were an embryo, your uterus, cervix, fallopian tubes, and vagina started out as two tubes that fused during your development within your mother's womb. The upper part of these two tubes remained separate and became your fallopian tubes. The center part of the two tubes fused to become your uterus, and the lower portion became the cervix and the upper vagina. A fusion defect, or uterine anomaly, may have developed along the way and your uterus, cervix, or upper vagina may not have fused completely or properly.

Two very distinct and separate groups of women are affected by uterine anomalies: women whose fusion defects are naturally occurring, and those whose defects were caused by their exposure to the synthetic hormone diethylstilbestrol (DES) while they were still in their mothers' wombs. (Ironically, DES, which came into common use in 1949 and was banned in 1971, was given to prevent miscarriage.) Twelve to 15 percent of women with recurrent abortions have a uterine anomaly, caused either by congenital defects or by DES exposure.

Congenital uterine anomalies occur in varying degrees, ranging from a complete reduplication of the uterus, cervix, and vagina—so that you have a doubling of everything—to mild fusion defects, such as the septate uterus.

Most of those who have congenital anomalies do well in pregnancy; indeed the woman may never know that she has such an anomaly. It's impossible to predict which women with the same malformation will do well in pregnancy and which will do poorly. There are no good statistics available because women who have malformations may not know it.

As a group, all women with congenital malformations have a 70 to 80 percent success rate once the malformation has been corrected, or the malformation has been diagnosed and the woman is carefully monitored. With certain congenital malformations, the chance of live birth increases with each subsequent pregnancy because the uterus goes through an adaptation process, due in part to mechanical stretching.

Women with DES malformations have a much poorer success rate since these malformations usually involve underdevelopment of the uterus and/or cervix. This underdevelopment cannot be corrected.

The Septate Uterus

Description: The septate uterus is a fusion defect that occurred when the uterus was being formed. A fibrous membrane, called a septum, extends into the uterus at the point where the fusion did not occur properly. The septum is generally avascular, meaning it has no blood vessels and, therefore, inhibits the growth of the placenta in that region. This inhibited placental growth could cause you to miscarry.

Symptoms: None until you try to get pregnant and miscarry repeatedly.

When the miscarriage happens: Usually in the first trimester, but sometimes in the second.

Miscarriage rate: For women with a large septum the miscarriage rate may approach 90 percent. Women with minor septums have close to normal reproductive potential. In fact, no good statistics on the incidence of septate uteri in the general population exist because it's believed that so many women with this fusion defect simply carry to term and, therefore, go undiagnosed.

Diagnosis: A test called a hysterosalpingogram will be performed by a radiologist. A small catheter will be placed into the cervix and an opaque dye will be injected under pressure into the uterine cavity. A series of films will be taken to see how the dye fills the uterine cavity, whether the dye travels through the tubes properly, and whether it goes out the ends of the fallopian tubes. The test takes about 45 minutes, and most women say it's quite uncomfortable, with moderate to severe menstrual cramping being experienced during the course of the procedure. No anesthetic is given.

Treatment: A surgical procedure called a hysteroscopic resection is performed under general anesthesia. It's done vaginally by either a reproductive endocrinologist or a gynecologist who has experience with this procedure.

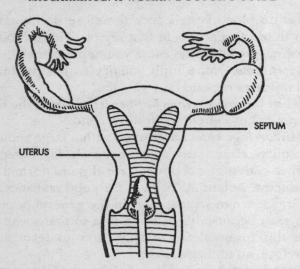

FIGURE 3. An example of a septate uterus. A fusion defect which occurs when the uterus is being formed results in a fibrous membrane called a septum extending into the uterus at the point where the fusion did not occur properly. The septum has few blood vessels and therefore inhibits the growth of the placenta in that region. This could cause miscarriage.

Your cervix will be dilated and your uterine cavity filled with a viscous solution to keep the walls of the cavity apart for the procedure. The doctor will insert a fiber-optic scope (hysteroscope) through which she will be able to see the uterine cavity. She will then use a resectoscope, a sharp instrument at the end of the fiber-optic scope, to shave off the septum and create a near normal uterine cavity. You'll go home the same day, after a few hours of observation for possible bleeding.

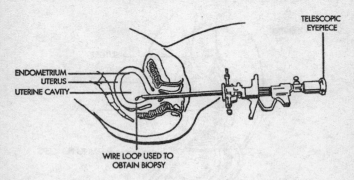

FIGURE 4. Hysteroscopy. The hysteroscope enables doctors to do a direct examination of the endometrium. The doctor inserts the lighted tip of the instrument through the vagina and cervix into the uterine cavity. There she can inspect any abnormal tissues and, using a tiny electrified loop, can even take samples for lab analysis.

Success rate: Although the success rate is 90 percent, it's worth noting that a woman with a corrected septate uterus will still be at an increased risk for problems in her subsequent pregnancies. She will be at high risk for preterm labor and delivery, and will usually require bed rest and intensive management of her pregnancy.

Because her uterus formed abnormally, it may not expand normally. This would cause increased pressure on the cervix, which, in turn, could cause it to dilate prematurely. Due to this premature dilating, women with a septate uterus may need a stitch in their cervix (called a *cerclage*) to help keep it closed when they are pregnant.

A cerclage is usually done on the labor floor of a

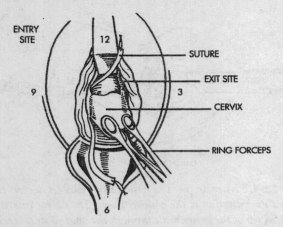

FIGURE 5a. The cerclage procedure. This figure shows placement of the first part of the stitch. The needle enters at 10 o'clock on the cervix and exits at 8 o'clock. The stitch is then brought under the cervix, re-enters the cervix at 4 o'clock and exits at 2 o'clock. The two loose ends are tied together, resulting in a circular loop that squeezes the cervix closed as seen in Figure 5b.

hospital under regional anesthesia. The upper and lower lip of the cervix are held with metal forceps and a stitch is placed circumferentially at the level where the cervix and the lower uterus meet. The suture is then tied tightly so that the cervix is closed. The stitch will be removed a few weeks before due date.

DES-Related Anomalies

Description: A misshapen or abnormally small uterus and, almost always, cervix. Usually the uterus is T-shaped and the cervix is hypoplastic, or under-

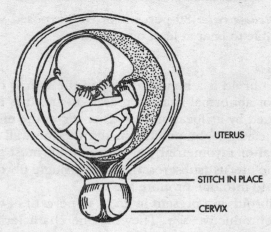

UTERUS

STITCH IN PLACE

CERVIX

FIGURE 5b. Internal view of the uterus after the cerclage procedure has been finished.

developed. This underdevelopment causes the cervix to be weak. It may dilate prematurely because it may not be able to maintain the pressure of the pregnancy well.

Frequency: About three million women received DES. Of their daughters, 50 to 80 percent will have some sort of uterine and/or cervical abnormality.

When the miscarriage happens: Usually in the first trimester, sometimes in the second.

Miscarriage rate: 40 percent.

Diagnosis: A hysterosalpingogram will be performed. (See explanation on page 57.)

Treatment: None, other than a cervical stitch (cerclage) and often bed rest for the duration of the pregnancy.

Success rate: 80 percent of DES-exposed women are able to bear at least one child.

Fibroids

A fibroid is a benign tumor of the uterus consisting of abnormal smooth muscle tissue. It is further defined by its location—whether it's in the endometrial cavity (submucous), in the uterine wall (intramural or myometrial), or on the outermost surface of the uterus (subserosal). Often a single fibroid will extend into one or more areas.

Fibroids are present in 25 to 40 percent of women of reproductive age. They may be characterized by excessive bleeding during or between periods, and pain or pressure. Most are asymptomatic.

Fibroids rarely cause miscarriage and should be considered a source of miscarriage only after all other possible causes have been ruled out. The vast majority of women who have fibroids conceive and carry to term without a problem. Pregnancies won't implant on fibroids because they're not a viable surface, and, in most people, pregnancies have ample room to grow around the fibroid.

The fibroids that would cause miscarriage are those that are usually submucous in location and are so large that they interfere with either implantation or the growth of the pregnancy.

In the small percentage of women in whom the fibroids are felt to be the source of recurrent pregnancy loss, their miscarriage rates can rise as high as 40 percent without treatment.

Miscarriages caused by fibroids occur either in the

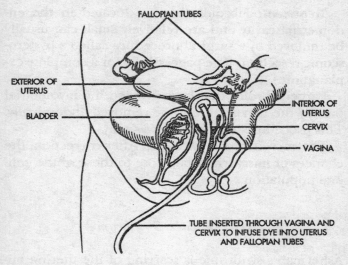

FIGURE 6. Hysterosalpingography. This procedure is used to help the doctor rule out the possibility of a physical barrier to conception. It is an X ray of the uterus and fallopian tubes. An opaque dye is infused by a narrow tube inserted through the vagina and cervix. The resulting pictures reveal any blockages in the egg's pathway through the fallopian tubes to successful implantation in the uterus.

first or second trimester. Fibroids are more often a source of pain and preterm uterine contractions in late pregnancy than a source of miscarriage.

Diagnosis: Many are detected during routine pelvic exams and by ultrasound. To identify the presence and location of submucous fibroids which may have bearing on a pregnancy a hysterosalpingogram will be performed. (See explanation on page 81.)

Treatment: Fibroids that are located in the endometrial cavity and are relatively small can usually be removed by a surgical procedure called a hysteroscopic resection. (See pages 81–84 for a complete explanation.)

Larger fibroids that have invaded the myometrial part of the uterus have to be removed abdominally. This procedure is called a *myomectomy*.

The success rate is excellent. After correction, the chances of miscarriage fall close to those of the general population.

Asherman's Syndrome

Asherman's syndrome is scarring of the uterine lining. It is rare but may be seen after a postpartum or postabortal uterine infection, or after a D&C done either for an incomplete abortion or for hemorrhaging after delivery. (Occasionally, in performing a D&C, the doctor strips away too much of the endometrial lining, resulting in a raw endometrial surface that will scar.)

A woman with minimal scarring may conceive and carry to term uneventfully; a woman with moderate scarring may miscarry; whereas a woman with severe scarring may be infertile and amenorrheic. Symptoms include absence of your period or much lighter menses than usual. You may have recurring pregnancy loss or infertility that developed after a D&C or a recent uterine infection.

Diagnosing Asherman's Syndrome

Diagnosis is made mostly by history. The doctor may suspect it when a patient reports the absence of menstruation following a D&C, or having a lighter than usual flow. The woman may give a history of fertility problems following a D&C.

If you have this kind of history, either a hysterosalpingogram or a hysteroscopy will be performed, depending on the level of suspicion. If your doctor is not sure if this is your problem, a hysterosalpingogram will be done by a radiologist. Scar tissue would be seen in areas where the dye didn't fill the uterus.

If your doctor is relatively certain that you have uterine scarring, she will probably diagnose it via hysteroscopy. The advantage of this method of diagnosis is that if the physician conducting the procedure sees scar tissue, she can eliminate it at the same time using a resectoscope. If she performs the surgery, the procedure is then called a hysteroscopic resection.

Treating Asherman's Syndrome

Some uterine walls will self-correct, but the majority will need a surgical procedure called a hysteroscopic resection. (See page 82 for a complete explanation.)

Sometimes, instead of a hysteroscopic resection, a D&C will be done to rescrape the uterine walls and, thereby, remove the scar tissue.

After either a hysteroscopic resection or a D&C, a catheter with a balloon at the end or an intrauterine device will be inserted into the uterus and the balloon will be inflated. This balloon will keep the uterine walls from touching each other, re-adhering, and scarring while your uterus heals.

After either of the above procedures, you'll be placed on a high dosage of estrogen for thirty days. The estrogen will build up the endometrial lining. For the last ten days of your treatment, you will also take progestin (synthetic progesterone). The progestin will trick your body into thinking you've ovulated and will bring on menstruation.

When the medication is stopped, the catheter with the balloon will be removed. You should get a normal period within a few days, indicating that your uterine lining was successfully rebuilt. If you don't get a period or it continues to be unusually light, the estrogen/progestin regimen will be repeated for one or two more cycles. It's unusual to need more than a second treatment course.

The treatment has a success rate of close to 100 percent. With treatment, the chance of miscarriage drops to the standard 20 percent as for the general population.

Incompetent Cervix

An incompetent cervix is too weak to support the increased pressure of a growing pregnancy. Some women with the condition never conceive, while in others the condition may be mistaken for preterm labor. The majority of incompetent cervices are idiopathic, which means we don't know why they are inherently weak.

Sometimes, an incompetent cervix is the result of DES exposure, or of obstetrical trauma, or of multiple second trimester abortions. The latter can cause your cervix to become incompetent because of the extent of surgical dilatation required to perform the termination. The cervix dilates just as much when you give birth, but there's something about the natural process occurring over hours and hours that keeps it from causing any lasting damage. When you perform second trimester termination, you're doing a mechanical dilatation to a cervix that doesn't have the hormonal milieu that it would have in full-term pregnancy.

When full term is reached, the cervix will usually have effaced and softened, having had a chance to change over time on its own. But in the second trimester, the cervix is firm, hard, and not in any way ready to dilate. An abortion at this stage forces it to dilate with instruments. As a result, the normal substance of the cervix may be broken down and may cause the cervix to be permanently damaged.

The extent to which a woman has to be dilated corresponds to the likelihood of her having a problem with her cervix in subsequent pregnancies. The later the termination and the more frequent, the greater the risk. An incompetent cervix accounts for 16 percent of second trimester losses. It is at this time that the weight of the pregnancy increases. Unless corrective measures are taken, each subsequent pregnancy will be lost earlier due to progressive weakening of the cervix.

Diagnosing an incompetent cervix

The cervix can appear completely normal in the nonpregnant state, or it may appear underdeveloped, as it does in many DES-exposed women. In more advanced cases, some suggestion of cervical dilatation may be noted in a pelvic exam in a nonpregnant state.

Unfortunately, the problem may not be diagnosed until you've lost a pregnancy. The typical scenario would be reaching the middle of your second trimester with your first pregnancy with no symptoms or hints of trouble until you feel a sensation of fullness in the vagina, which is usually either the membranes bulging through the cervix or the pregnancy starting to protrude. At this point it is usually too late to save the pregnancy. Your next pregnancy should be followed with frequent pelvic exams and treatment, if necessary. If you've had a pregnancy loss and this condition is suspected, your doctor may perform a hysterosalpingogram to determine if your cervix is dilated in the nonpregnant state.

Treating an incompetent cervix

A cerclage or cervical stitch will be put in toward the end of your first trimester or the beginning of the second. You will be placed on complete bed rest for the rest of your pregnancy. This treatment has a success rate of 80 percent.

INFECTIOUS ORGANISMS

Most infections are one-time, sporadic events. The only infectious organisms thought possibly to play a role in recurrent miscarriages are *mycoplasma* and *ureaplasma*.

Mycoplasma and ureaplasma are part of some women's normal vaginal flora. They're common in the general population but are seen more often in populations with infertility and with higher miscarriage rates. These organisms seem to play a role in miscarriage, but how they do so is not yet known. The organisms are often asymptomatic. They are diagnosed by vaginal culture.

Tetracycline is prescribed for both the woman and her partner if she's not pregnant. Erythromycin is prescribed for the woman if she is pregnant. Treatment should reduce her miscarriage rate to that of the general population if the infection can be effectively eradicated.

CHROMOSOMAL ABNORMALITIES

Unlike the chromosomal abnormalities that occur randomly, in these cases one or both parents are carrying some kind of chronically defective genetic material, which accounts for 3 to 8 percent of recurrent miscarriages.

Many different kinds of chromosomal aberrations

can be carried by parents, and many of them are not diagnosable. Of the known recurrent abnormalities, the one that most commonly causes miscarriage is called a *balanced translocation*.

When you have a balanced translocation, two chromosomes break and rejoin incorrectly. This means that one chromosome ends up carrying too much genetic information, and one ends up carrying too little. A balanced translocation can happen as a sporadic event, or it can be passed down from one of the parents to the fetus. Women are twice as likely to carry a balanced translocation as are men.

The parent who has these kinds of genes functions normally. But when she or he attempts to have children, problems can occur unless the two chromosome pairs align properly. If this does not occur, the fetus will end up with either too much or too little genetic information and will miscarry, usually in the first eight weeks.

For example, let's say that in the mother, part of chromosome 13 is attached to chromosome 14 and part of 14 reciprocally joins 13. She contains all her normal genetic material, it's just in the wrong places. She functions normally and appears normal because she has all her genes. However, when she tries to have children and her chromosomes double and split, if the newly formed 13/14 chromosome doesn't match up with the reciprocal 14/13 chromosome, the pregnancy is going to end up with either too much or too little genetic information and will miscarry. However, if the chromosomes align correctly, that pregnancy will be normal, barring any other un-related chromosomal abnormalities, and the fetus will carry this translocation.

At any given time only 33 percent of the pregnancies will receive the proper balance of chromosomes. The other 67 percent will have mismatches where they have too little or too much genetic material, and will miscarry. Many of these conceptions escape detection as they end soon after fertilization.

Diagnosing Chromosomal Abnormalities

Sometimes the problem is found during amniocentesis. If you've miscarried, the diagnosis is generally made via testing of the aborted material and then confirmed by *karyotypes* on the parents. A karyotype maps out the chromosomal structure in both parents. It's done by taking blood from the parents and doing a chromosome analysis of their white blood cells and observing the patterns they form. It takes about a week for the results.

One of the ironies of testing a woman for chromosomal abnormalities is that the diagnostic procedures can, in rare cases, cause miscarriages. Amniocentesis and chronic villi sampling, two invasive and relatively crude procedures, trigger miscarriages in a small percentage of pregnant women. That risk is diminished with a revolutionary procedure developed in 1996 that uses a simple blood sample drawn from a woman's arm. Physicians have known since the 1960s that a tiny number of fetal cells cross the placenta and wind up in the mother's bloodstream; the new test, the equivalent of finding a fetal needle in the mother's haystack, finds these cells and analyzes them.

If you must have amniocentesis, you can reduce your risk of miscarriage by making sure the test is not performed before the fifteenth week of pregnancy. Women who have this procedure earlier are 11 times more likely to miscarry, according to 1996 research at the University of Alabama at Birmingham. In the study, women who had the earlier amnios were about 15 times more likely to leak amniotic fluid and about 10 times more likely to experience vaginal bleeding, compared to women who had the procedure at the normal fifteenth to eighteenth week. Both complications heighten the risk for miscarriage.

Treating Chromosomal Abnormalities

You will be told that you will have to go through a lot of pregnancy loss in order to have a family. There is no treatment readily available at present. *Note:* All the other malformations that can occur when chromosomes are passed on to the fetus basically work in a similar manner. If they match up properly, the fetus is normal. If they don't, you'll miscarry. The success rate is the same for all of them.

A new area of research involves pre-implantation chromosomal analysis. With this technique, following in vitro fertilization, a cell from the developing zygote is analyzed. If it carries the appropriate chromosomal complement, it is implanted in the mother.

Finally, a new procedure may allow physicians to screen a woman's eggs before in vitro fertilization, weeding out those with abnormal chromosomes. This technique, announced in 1996 by Dr. Santiago Munne of Saint Barnabas Medical Center in Orange, New Jersey, could benefit women who suffer repeated miscarriages because a substantial proportion of their eggs carry chromosomal abnormalities. It could also help older women, because aging eggs typically develop such abnormalities over time.

Antiphospholipid Syndrome

Antiphospholipid syndrome is an autoimmune syndrome that accounts for 10 to 15 percent of recurrent miscarriages, usually occurring in the first or second trimester.

Normally, your immune system produces different types of antibodies to fight off various toxins and infections. People with autoimmune syndromes and/or diseases produce antibodies to their own tissues or cells. These types of antibodies are called *autoantibodies*. A syndrome refers to a group of findings that do not mean the same thing all the time. In other words, the presence of these autoantibodies will not affect everyone in the same way.

People with antiphospholipid syndrome (APLS) produce autoantibodies to phospholipids, which are fatty molecules on the cell membranes. For reasons that are still unknown, these autoantibodies cause blood clots to form. These blood clots may develop anywhere in the body. If they form in the blood vessels of the placenta, the fetus will be deprived of oxygen and nutrients. If these clots are mild, they will lead to growth retardation. If severe, they will lead to the loss of the pregnancy. It is the extent of clot formation that determines the severity of the disease.

APLS was discovered and linked with miscarriage in 1983. It was originally called anticardiolipin syndrome. Cardiolipin is a type of phospholipid, and it was the first such compound associated with this syndrome. The name of the syndrome was changed when researchers realized that other phospholipids are also involved.

The presence of the autoantibody anticardiolipin in your blood is required in order for you to be officially diagnosed as having APLS. However, the presence of another substance—a protein called *lupus anticoagulant*—will result in the same type of blood clotting and pregnancy complications.

All normal, healthy people continually make blood clots and then break them down. Lupus anticoagulant prevents the proper breakdown of blood clots, and this results in increased clotting. Lupus anticoagulant can be present in the blood either alone or in conjunction with anticardiolipin. While the presence of lupus anticoagulant alone will not give you an official diagnosis of APLS, you may be treated in the same manner as if you did have the syndrome.

Those with an autoimmune disease such as thyroid disease, lupus, or rheumatoid arthritis are more likely to have anticardiolipins and/or lupus anticoagulants in their blood. Having one of these autoimmune diseases does not mean that you definitely *do* have lupus anticoagulants and/or anticardiolipins. The chances that you might are simply higher. However, you may also have lupus anticoagulants and anticardiolipins in your blood even if you don't have an autoimmune disease.

Symptoms of APLS

Unfortunately, the main symptom of APLS is recurrent pregnancy loss. Until they get pregnant, many women with APLS are often healthy and symptom-free. Sometimes, however, blood clots may form in other parts of the body, and these may produce symptoms. For instance, if the blood clots form in the brain, you might have ministrokes. If the blood clots travel to the lungs, you may have difficulty breathing. If the clots travel to your heart, you may have a heart attack. Such presentations are rare in the reproductive-age woman, but women with these factors must be followed carefully throughout their lifetimes.

Obtaining an APLS diagnosis

You will be sent for a blood test and your blood will be screened for both lupus anticoagulant and anticardiolipins as well as several other factors associated with the coagulation process (these include antithrombin III, protein C, and protein S). These will be measured in units called titers, which show how strong the antibody response is. The higher your titer, the more of an immune response you're creating and the higher the likelihood that you will have a problem with your pregnancy. It's impossible to say exactly what level of antibodies would be harmful because everyone's reaction to these substances is different.

Treatment of APLS

The higher your titer, the more aggressive your treatment will be. You will definitely take one baby aspirin daily to thin your blood. Your doctor may also prescribe heparin, a stronger blood thinner, and the steroid prednisone. Prednisone suppresses the immune system and is given to organ transplant patients to keep their bodies from rejecting the new organ. Prednisone is being used less frequently because doctors are seeing equally good success rates with baby aspirin and heparin alone.

There are a few side effects, however. The aspirin and heparin will alter your ability to form clots. This is significant if you cut yourself or need to have surgery. Long-term heparin use results in demineralization of bone, which can lead to osteoporosis. Prednisone can have severe side effects. It can cause you to become depressed, you may retain fluid, and you will be more prone to many infections since it suppresses your immune system.

If you're diagnosed as having antiphospholipid syndrome, your obstetrician will refer you to a perinatalogist, a high-risk pregnancy specialist, who will then either take over your treatment or work in conjunction with your obstetrician. Treatment should begin before conception or as soon as the pregnancy is confirmed. The success rate is between 70 to 80 percent.

Note: If you have antiphospholipid syndrome, your

pregnancy will have to be monitored very carefully for late pregnancy complications. You will have an increased risk of preeclampsia and fetal growth retardation. Preeclampsia is a disorder unique to pregnancy characterized by hypertension, edema, and protein in the urine. It is usually seen in third trimester and can lead to seizures, coma, and loss of life if untreated. After delivery you may be placed on anticoagulating medication for life.

Now let's turn our attention to a more recent development that has brought to light other causes of recurring miscarriages, conditions of which you—and possibly even your obstetrician—may not be aware.

A RECENT BREAKTHROUGH

In the early 1980s great strides began to be made in the field of immunology, and researchers discovered a defect in a mother's immune system that accounts for some of those previously unexplained miscarriages.

Researchers have come up with treatments for the defects that have close to an 80 percent success rate. Further investigation of the defects continues, and the methods of treating them are expected to improve even more.

Ongoing research in immunology is expected to find other causes of recurring miscarriages, bringing even more hope to women whose reasons for recurrent miscarriage are still labeled "unknown."

Deficiency of Fetal-Blocking Antibodies

In order for the mother to protect her fetus, she has to create fetal-blocking antibodies, which, as the name suggests, block her other antibodies from recognizing the fetus as foreign and destroying it. A deficiency of fetal-blocking antibodies accounts for 10 percent or less of recurring miscarriages.

The cue to produce fetal-blocking antibodies comes from a substance in the cells called *histocompatibility locus antigen* (HLA). An antigen is a component of a cell that can stimulate the creation of antibodies in your body if the antigen is recognized as something foreign. For example, if a kidney with antigens different from yours was transplanted into your body, an immune response would be stimulated to try to rid the body of the "foreign" kidney. When medical centers search for compatible donors for organ transplants, that's what they're screening for—someone with as many matching antigens as possible.

When a sperm penetrates an egg, it carries in antigens that are different from yours, but it also carries in histocompatibility locus antigens. The fertilizing sperm's HLA merges with your HLA, causing your body to create the blocking antibodies that will protect the pregnancy. Problems arise when the father's and mother's HLAs are too similar. The signal to produce the blocking antibodies will then be very weak, not enough blocking antibodies will be produced, and your body will recognize as "foreign" all the other antigens that the sperm brought with it to the pregnancy. Your body will destroy those foreign antigens, thereby destroying the pregnancy.

Obtaining a Diagnosis and Treatment for a Deficiency

Obstetricians are beginning to accept the fact that a lack of fetal-blocking antibodies exists as a medical condition, but screening for the condition is still being conducted only by the two main research centers studying the condition.

Since standard testing is not available, you will be sent to one of the few medical centers researching this condition for treatment.

At these centers, you will receive an injection of your husband's or a donor's white blood cells to stimulate an immune response against those cells. The theory behind this treatment is that while your HLA is similar, it is not identical, and the amount of HLA carried in by the sperm is not enough to trigger an immune response in your body. However, if you're injected with a larger amount of HLA, which is what's happening when you're being injected with your husband's white blood cells, then that larger amount of HLA will stimulate an immune response. In effect, you're being immunized against your husband's HLA. The next time you get pregnant, you will have an immune response to the HLA, and you will form the fetal-blocking antibodies. Although this treatment is controversial it is reportedly successful 80 percent of the time.

EVALUATING FUTURE FINDINGS

As for other causative factors, you may hear news reports about something that isn't mentioned in this book; perhaps you'll hear about yet another study saying caffeine is harmful to your pregnancy, followed by one that says it isn't.

Here are some good criteria to apply to help you judge the validity of medical studies you hear or read about:

▼ What medical journal first published the study? *The New England Journal of Medicine, The Lancet, The Journal of the American Medical Association, Obstetrics and Gynecology,* and *The American Journal of Obstetrics and Gynecology* are the most reputable journals. They accept and publish the best designed and, therefore, most reliable studies.

▼ Where was the study conducted? The bigger and more reliable the institution, usually the bigger and more reliable the study.

▼ How many people did the study follow? A group of five is much less applicable to the general population than if a group of thousands was studied.

Ideally, if you have any questions or concerns about a new finding, ask your doctor about it.

Participating in a Research Study

Research into other causes of recurrent miscarriages is always being conducted at universities across the country. To find a study near you, ask your obstetrician or reproductive endocrinologist (a specialist in recurrent pregnancy loss) to refer you to a teaching institution where research is taking place.

If your doctor is unable to help you, go to a medical library and look up the diagnosis that you have—or simply look up the topic of recurrent miscarriage—to see where the most research is being conducted. Call that institution and ask for a referral in your geographic area.

You may also contact the department of obstetrics and gynecology at a major academic institution in your area and ask the department chairman's office for information on any research study that may be ongoing or about to start.

THE OTHER 25 PERCENT

Seventy-five percent of the women who have repeatedly miscarried will have been miscarrying due to one of the causes we've mentioned so far. The other 25 percent, unfortunately, will come to the end of their workups with no diagnosable reason. If you fall into this category two things are recommended:

▼ Taking clomiphene citrate. This should be done on the assumption that maybe you *do* have a luteal phase defect, but you just happened to have a nondiagnostic biopsy.

▼ A course of tetracycline between pregnancies for

both the woman and the man to rid the body of any possible undiagnosed infection of mycoplasma or ureaplasma, which can have false negative readings on their cultures.

THE EFFECTS OF STRESS

Stress is difficult to measure because it affects everyone in different ways, but it may have a deleterious effect on one's health and therefore one's reproductive potential.

One massive 1998 study involving 16,000 in seventeen European countries suggests that workplace stress can increase your chances of giving birth prematurely, especially if the work demands long hours and you don't like your job. Similarly, occupational health specialists at the University of California at Davis found that lawyers who worked long hours on the job were three times as likely to miscarry as were those who worked fewer than thirty-five hours a week.

If you're repeatedly miscarrying and feel anxious or stressed on a daily basis, it would be worthwhile to talk to a psychotherapist about how better to cope with daily stress.

Now that we've discussed the physical aspects of miscarriage, it's time to turn to the emotional aspects of losing a pregnancy. In the next chapter, we will discuss what you can expect from the mourning process and how even well-intentioned friends and family members may complicate this process for you by saying the wrong things or coming across as unempathetic. We'll tell you how to handle this—and other situations that may arise—during various stages of your grieving process.

5

▼

THE MOURNING
AFTER

Miscarriage is a loss that, like any other, needs to be mourned properly. Otherwise, your feelings of grief will remain trapped inside and may later come out in negative ways, such as lingering depression or anger directed at inappropriate people or situations.

Mourning a miscarriage is more complex than any other type of mourning because there was no tangible object for the grief that has been generated. You never had a chance to meet your baby. Your doctor and your friends and family may be discounting your grief. Perhaps they're telling you just to have another baby. By being so focused on the future—and not on your loss—they're probably making you wonder if your feelings are appropriate.

The most important thing for you to keep in mind
as you read this chapter is that there is no right or
wrong way for you to feel after a miscarriage. As long
as you have no desire to hurt yourself or others, *any-*
thing you're feeling is all right. However, if at any
point in your grieving process you find yourself wanting to harm either yourself or others, seek psychological counseling immediately. Ask your obstetrician
for a referral to a therapist specializing in pregnancy
loss, or request a referral from one of the sources
listed at the end of this book.

As you read on, remember that mourning is a
unique experience, as individual as you are. No two
people will grieve in exactly the same way.

No matter how you're grieving, we hope this chapter will help you as you go through this difficult but
necessary process.

WHY A MISCARRIAGE IS SO DIF-
FICULT TO MOURN

Few obstetricians acknowledge a woman's need to
mourn a miscarriage. Most physicians downplay the
emotional significance of miscarriage by saying things
like "It's no big deal," "It's a natural part of pregnancy," and "It happens to everyone."

This can make you feel your grief is inappropriate
and, because of that feeling, you'll have trouble dealing with it. But there are also other reasons for this
trouble. There are three factors that make grieving
any loss more difficult, and all three apply to miscar-

riage, according to clinical psychologist Ruth S. Jacobs, Ph.D., who is on the advisory board of Miscarriage, Infant Death and Stillbirth (MIDS), an Englewood, N.J.–based support group, and who has personally suffered two stillbirths. These three factors are:

1. *Suddenness:* This makes grieving harder, says Jacobs, because you didn't have time to prepare for your loss. "People have had plenty of time to prepare for what they wanted the baby to be like, for their hopes and their dreams," she says. "If you don't have time to prepare for your loss, it will take you longer to adjust to it."

2. *Untimeliness:* "One expects pregnancy to go for nine months," says Jacobs. "When it ends after a certain number of weeks, it's like a child who dies out of turn. The untimeliness of this loss often causes the woman to spend lots of time thinking, 'That wasn't supposed to happen' and, especially in cases where no definite cause is given for the miscarriage, to start blaming herself for it. She spends a lot of time thinking, 'If only I'd done X, Y, or Z, maybe the baby would be alive.' "

3. *Ambiguity:* After a miscarriage, there is no object for the grief that has been generated. There is no baby to hold, no baby to bury, no baby to remember. "You've never met this child, and so you're not mourning a concrete person," says Jacobs. "Obviously, mourning someone you've never met is much more complicated than mourning someone who was a part of your life. You're mourning hopes and dreams, which is a much more difficult

thing to mourn than when you've actually known a person and you have memories of them."

What Friends and Family Say, or Don't Say

As if it weren't already hard enough to mourn a miscarriage, your friends and family will probably make it even harder for you by minimizing your loss or not talking about it.

"One of the most difficult things for couples going through a miscarriage is that people don't recognize it as a real loss," says Jacobs. "Instead of acknowledging it by saying, 'I'm so sorry for your loss,' people minimize it by saying well-intentioned but unhelpful things like, 'You're young, you'll have another one' or 'It wasn't meant to be' or 'It's God's will' or 'At least you know you're fertile.' Hearing those kinds of things will only make the couple hold onto the baby longer and say, 'But that was a real baby, that was my baby even if I have a hundred other babies.' They want the loss to be validated, and the more society minimizes the loss, the more the person is likely to hold onto the loss and not be able to work it through."

HOW TO MAKE THE MOURNING A LITTLE EASIER

So what should you do when someone minimizes your loss or doesn't bring it up after a certain period of time has passed, and they think you should be over it? You should raise the subject yourself if you feel the need to, says Jacobs. (Generally, others will tend to feel that after two weeks of being upset you should be over your grief. In reality, it takes most women anywhere from three months to a year to recover emotionally from a miscarriage.)

As for comments that minimize your loss, she recommends saying something like, "I know that you mean well, but what you're saying to me is not helpful to me." Then tell them, "You can do or say X, Y, or Z instead."

Educating Others

Many women feel that their friends and family should automatically be more empathetic, but, the truth is, until people have experienced miscarriage themselves, they simply don't understand what a wrenching loss it is. They don't know that the things they're saying to you aren't helpful. "They need to be educated," says Jacobs. "Although this puts the grieving couple in the unfortunate position of having another burden—that of educating the public—I think that's the only way a couple will actually get what they need from their friends and family, and that is the only way their friends and family will learn what they need to do. A couple will often say nothing when someone has minimized their loss because they don't want to make the other person feel bad. Meanwhile, the person who's supposed to be doing the comforting is making the couple feel worse. There's something wrong with that picture, and it has to be reversed for the sake of everyone involved."

Helping Yourself

Sometimes, however, the people in your life just won't be able to give you what you need. In those instances, Jacobs recommends doing one or more of the following, depending on what feels right for you:

Read about the Subject

Why is reading helpful? "You could start to feel crazy if you're mourning and other people are making you feel like it's wrong to be doing so. Reading will help you understand that it's okay, it's *healthy*, to mourn," says Jacobs. "Reading will also help you know that other people have been through what you're going through. This will make you feel less isolated when your friends or your family let you down. The isolation and the feeling that you're the only one that this has happened to—a feeling that arises because society simply doesn't talk about miscarriage, because society engages in what I call a conspiracy of silence—make it harder to grieve. Knowing what you can expect and knowing that you're not crazy can really cut down on the length of the mourning process."

Join a Support Group

This serves the same function as reading. It helps validate your feelings and lets you know that other people have gone through similar experiences. (See Appendix I for a list of support groups.)

Hold a Memorial Service or Enact Some Sort of a Ritual

"This is a way of providing closure the way a funeral provides closure," says Jacobs. "Rituals that have helped people include lighting candles, making donations in memory of the baby, writing a poem or in a journal, or planting flowering bushes." Any ritual is fine. The most important thing is that it feels right to you and your partner.

Hormonal Changes After a Miscarriage

After a miscarriage you will experience a significant drop in estrogen, which will affect your mood for two to six weeks after your miscarriage, depending on the gestational age at which you miscarried. However, don't think that any sadness you're feeling over the miscarriage is strictly hormonally based. You are experiencing appropriate grief that is augmented by your drop in estrogen. This drop will exacerbate your underlying mental state, but keep in mind that even after your estrogen level has reverted to normal, your feelings of sadness may continue.

THE STAGES OF GRIEF

Most women who experience miscarriage define it as
a death and mourn it as such. After a death, people
often think their grieving will follow a set course.
They think there are specific stages they will go
through, and that eventually they'll reach the final
stage and will know in a clear-cut way that they are
over their grief. But that's not the way it happens.

"It's important to realize that we don't go from
stage one to stage two to stage three," says Sharon
Covington, M.S.W., a clinical social worker who is in
private practice and is also the director of counseling
for the Shady Grove Fertility Center in Rockville,
Maryland, and is on the advisory board for SHARE-
Pregnancy and Infant Loss Support, Inc. She herself
suffered one miscarriage and two early stillbirths and
started a self-help support group in Washington,
D.C., called MIS—Miscarriage Infant Death and Stillbirth. "There are no cookbook recipes for grieving.
It's a very personal experience based upon people's
personalities and life experiences.

"Grief is like a tidal wave that sweeps over you," she
says. "The feelings of shock and disbelief are followed by many different kinds of feelings, including
anger, guilt, and depression. Those feelings grow
and crest with time. They seem to peak for people
somewhere between three to nine months following
the loss. But it's important for people to know that
grief occurs in a somewhat unpredictable and repeti-
tive way. Even after it's peaked and begun to ebb,
grief will recur. I call these recurring feelings "swells

of grief," which are the same feelings but not of the same magnitude. These swells can be touched off by many different things. We all have our own triggers. They can be the due date, the anniversary of the miscarriage, a song, a holiday like Mother's Day or Father's Day. Finally, grief never fully goes away. It lingers as a shadow, as a sense that in some ways this loss will be in your heart forever, but it's no longer going to take the same kind of energy to deal with the feelings that loss elicits."

The stages of grief that most people associate with death were established for the dying person by Elisabeth Kübler-Ross in 1969 in her book *On Death and Dying*. They apply to the bereaved as well and are as follows:

1. Denial
2. Anger
3. Bargaining
4. Depression
5. Acceptance

All of these stages apply to the mourning of a miscarriage, except for bargaining since there's nothing you can try to do—no good deed you can pledge or negative character trait you can change—to prevent a miscarriage. Unlike people who have time to prepare for a death, your mourning will begin once the miscarriage is over. Therefore, the four stages you can expect to deal with are the same as Kübler-Ross's, minus the bargaining stage. You will feel some or all of the following stages in your own unique order. You may not feel all of them and that's okay because your grief is as unique as you are.

Denial

As was mentioned earlier, the life changes most difficult to adjust to are those that happen suddenly, catching us unaware and unprepared. Few things happen more suddenly than a miscarriage. One day you're pregnant, and the next day you're not. Because of this suddenness it's common for women to experience an emotional response lag—a state of numbness during which their emotions have not yet caught up to reality. For a few weeks after the miscarriage you may feel stunned and unable to believe what has happened. Everything around you may take on a slight tinge of unreality.

The shock and denial experienced during this period "serve the purpose or giving you some opportunity to begin to psychologically adjust to the magnitude of what's happened," says Covington. You will probably get through the weeks immediately following your miscarriage by doing what's expected of you. On automatic pilot, you'll take care of your husband and the house and may return to work just days after the miscarriage. You'll function just as you functioned before, sometimes better because you desperately need to fulfill your daily responsibilities as a way of numbing your pain.

But denial lasts only so long. Next comes anger.

Anger

Most people think of anger as a negative emotion, but feeling angry about the fact that miscarriage happened to you and not to the pregnant woman next door is actually very healthy since it is a sign that you have begun to accept your loss as a reality. You can't be angry at something unless you accept the fact that it has happened. This coming to terms with reality and the anger generated by this step is a necessary part of moving forward and working through your grief.

Most women have a hard time dealing with anger since most of us have been raised to feel that anger is a bad emotion, one that should not be expressed. Nothing could be further from the truth. If you don't let out your anger it will "sit there and fester," writes grief counselor Helen Fitzgerald in *The Mourning Handbook,* "growing larger and larger until it erupts. Anger that is not discharged can create both emotional and physical stress leading to anxiety and depression. Anger that is not acknowledged and that is misdirected can create all sorts of problems in your life. It is healthier, both physically and emotionally, to learn to identify your [angry] feelings and express them appropriately."

The anger stage is a very difficult one, since anger often doesn't show itself in clear-cut ways. During this stage you may feel you're going crazy as you struggle to deal with confused feelings and crying jags that may occur at unexpected times in unexpected places. Seeing pregnant women or women with children may bring on strong feelings of sadness or jealousy. This sadness and jealousy are really manifestations of anger over the fact that it seems as if everybody else in the world can have babies except you.

At this point you may feel that you're losing control of yourself. You want to mourn but, chances are, you're being made to feel that mourning is inappropriate. You're angry, but you're not quite sure what you're angry about or whom you're angry at. Unfortunately, you will probably be ready to deal with your feelings of anger at a time when your friends and family will be thinking that you should already be getting over your loss. Because they may not be giving you the support you need, you may find yourself channeling your feelings of anger toward them. Keep in mind that while you may indeed be angry at your friends and family for letting you down, what you're mostly angry about is the fact that you lost your baby. You're probably angry at how your feelings of joy over being pregnant were so abruptly snatched away from you. If the miscarriage happened during your first pregnancy, you may be angry at the fact that it will never be that special first time ever again.

How to Handle Your Anger

"Anger creates a rush of energy that can get out of hand and cause you to do or say things that you will be sorry for later," writes Fitzgerald. "It is important to recognize [when you are angry] and to have ways to discharge this destructive energy In appropriate ways."

The steps Fitzgerald recommends for releasing the energy created by anger include such physical activities as brisk walking, a fast-paced sport, hitting a punching bag, or cleaning your house. If your anger brings out a need to destroy, she recommends having things around that can be destroyed such as old telephone books you can tear up. In short, do whatever works for you. If writing a letter or writing in your journal helps you get in touch with, and release, your angry feelings, then by all means do that. If talking to your husband or a friend who is really open to listening to what you're feeling works for you, then go that route. You know yourself best. Do whatever you can to help yourself feel your anger and get it out of your system.

Guilt and Blame

Feeling guilty is not an official stage of grieving, but it is something that most women will be feeling now, particularly if they weren't given a reason for their miscarriage. They will often start blaming themselves for the miscarriage and wonder what they could have done to prevent it.

How to Handle Your Guilt and Blame

If you find you're blaming yourself for your miscarriage, it's time for you to call or pay another visit to your doctor. You last saw her or him during a time of crisis, and you surely didn't have as many questions for the doctor as you do now. You've probably done some reading about the causes of miscarriage. You know that some women miscarry not because of random chromosomal problems with the pregnancy but because of something that is wrong with their own bodies. Knowing this, you may incorrectly start diagnosing yourself, convinced that if only this or that condition had been discovered, you would still be carrying your baby.

Your doctor may allay your feelings of guilt by telling you that your miscarriage had nothing to do with your health, your husband's health, or with anything that you did. If she tells you that you didn't do anything to cause your miscarriages, believe her.

Depression

People tend to think of depression as an illness, but feeling depressed is a perfectly healthy part of the grief process. "The depression one may experience over the death of a loved one can last for an hour, a day, a week or longer," writes Fitzgerald. "It is normal to feel depressed after a major loss in your life. The severity or longevity will vary from person to person."

She lists the basic symptoms of depression as including some or all of the following:

▼ Not caring about your appearance
▼ Never changing your clothes
▼ Withdrawing from friends and activities

▼ Low self-esteem
▼ Lack of confidence
▼ Negative attitudes about everything
▼ Feeling empty inside
▼ Lacking energy
▼ Shedding tears at the slightest provocation
▼ Lacking interest in anything, including sex
▼ Weight gain or weight loss
▼ Insomnia or excessive sleep
▼ Feeling overwhelmed by ordinary daily tasks

How to Handle Your Depression

Know that it's normal to feel depressed and know that this painful stage is going to pass with time. As with anger, do whatever you can to help you get in touch with and express your feelings of depression.

Covington recommends that you find ways to talk about it, either with your partner, with friends, in a support group, or in a journal. Getting your feelings of depression out is important because, as Covington says, "a feeling shared is a feeling diminished."

While you're feeling depressed, it's important that you take good physical care of yourself. Eating right, exercising, and getting plenty of sleep will all help you be better able to cope with your depression and to get over it more quickly.

However, if your depression lingers for more than two weeks, or if it becomes so overwhelming that your day-to-day functioning is impaired, or if you have thoughts of suicide, you should seek professional help immediately.

ACCEPTANCE

In this stage, you no longer deny reality, no longer feel angry about it, and you no longer feel depressed about it. Of course, you'll still feel sad from time to time, but it won't be that overwhelming, all-encompassing feeling of depression you experienced in the previous stage.

In *The Mourning Handbook,* Fitzgerald lists a number of things to help you recognize that you're well on your way to accepting your loss. Some that are appropriate to miscarriage include:

▼ Being in touch with the finality of your loss
▼ Being able to enjoy time alone
▼ Being able to drive somewhere by yourself without crying the whole time
▼ Realizing that painful comments made by family or friends were made in ignorance
▼ Looking forward to holidays
▼ Being able to reach out to help someone in a similar situation
▼ Having your eating, sleeping, and exercise patterns return to what they were before
▼ No longer feeling tired all the time
▼ Being able to concentrate on a book or a favorite television program
▼ Discovering personal growth as a result of your loss

Only once you experience most of the above will you be emotionally ready to conceive again.

When to Seek Professional Help

If your ever feel that you don't want to live, that you want to join your baby, you should get help immediately.

Other signs that professional help may benefit you are if any of the following occur at a time when you feel your intensity of mourning should be easing:

▼ Getting stuck in any of the normal stages of grief. For example, if you're angry all the time or continue to blame yourself for the miscarriage, or if your depression worsens or doesn't lift.

▼ Inappropriate behavior at inappropriate times, such as crying for no reason or feeling very angry but not knowing where your anger is coming from. This can be a sign that you've suppressed your feelings over the loss of your pregnancy and may need help coming to terms with them and working them through.

▼ Finding yourself unable to enjoy life or get along with other people.

▼ Not being able to fulfill your daily responsibilities.

▼ Not being able to get out of bed.

▼ Not eating correctly.

▼ Insomnia.

▼ Thinking about the miscarriage all the time.

▼ Needing more support than your friends or family are able to give you.

▼ Feeling that you need professional help.

If any of the above apply to you, ask your obstetrician, your hospital social work department, or your local pregnancy loss support group to recommend a therapist who specializes in pregnancy loss.

MISCARRIAGE AND YOUR MARRIAGE

Like any other crisis, a miscarriage will bring out the cracks in a relationship. Sometimes, these cracks may be too large to mend. In an otherwise good marriage, however, much of the trouble that couples experience after a miscarriage is the result of misunderstanding each other, and can be avoided if you keep a few things in mind.

First, Covington says, it's important for you to remember that you bonded differently with the baby than your husband did. "Research has shown that women's and men's sense of bonding and attachment isn't equal until around the time of the birth," she says, "and the time where there's the biggest difference in bonding is in early pregnancy. Just as you bonded differently, you will grieve differently. It's very important for couples to know that they're going to feel and deal differently with that and to be able to allow each other to do that."

Secondly, keep in mind that, as Jacobs explains, after a miscarriage, sex-role stereotypes get perpetuated. The wife is expected to grieve. The man is socialized to go back to work and not ask about his own feelings. Inside, the woman may feel like a failure as a woman because she miscarried. The man may feel like a failure as a man because he was not able to protect his wife from the miscarriage and the ensuing emotional pain it caused her.

Husbands tend to think they have to solve all of their wives' problems.

Understand Each Other's Ways of Grieving

Conflict often arises between husbands and wives because most husbands, in an effort to support their wives emotionally, tend to keep their own feelings about the miscarriage to themselves. Their wives, in turn, take their silence to mean that their husbands don't care about what has happened—both to the baby and to them.

So what's a couple to do? They should openly tell each other how they are feeling and simply listen to each other without judging or telling each other they shouldn't be feeling that way. "It's a mistake," Jacobs warns, "for each to believe that the other should experience what he or she is experiencing and that things will be okay only if they're both feeling the same thing."

Women "need to be sensitized" to how their husbands are mourning, says Jacobs. "It might be different from the way they are mourning, but it doesn't mean they take the loss any less seriously or that it's any reflection on the state of the marriage. It's usually more a reflection on the way men and women are socialized. If women and men become aware of those differences, then they can work through them. If they don't become aware of the differences, then they'll become more isolated and more withdrawn from each other, and that will perpetuate the conflict."

Keep the Lines of Communication Open

What can you do to ease the strain or distance you may be feeling in your marriage?

"Talk," says Covington. "Sometimes it helps to set a time limit on these conversations. Agree that you'll talk about it for ten or twenty minutes every day, and at the end of that time put the subject aside until the next day. What sometimes happens is that husbands may be afraid to talk to their wives about the miscarriage because they're afraid that once that conversation starts it's never going to stop. Putting a boundary on the time you spend talking about it will make it more manageable for him."

Another reason your husband may be reluctant to talk about the miscarriage is because he may think you expect him to fix things. Men are often under the misconception that you want them to do something about the problem, when all you really want to do is to cry and for him to allow you to do that. But your crying often perpetuates his feeling of inadequacy. If this is happening in your marriage, tell your husband straight out: "Look, I don't want you to fix this. I just want you to let me cry on your shoulder." Chances are he'll let you do that, and this will make both of you feel closer to each other. You'll be able to express your feelings, and he'll know he's giving you what you need, which is his shoulder to cry on.

If your husband continues to be unable to deal with your grief, or if he doesn't seem to be grieving himself, Jacobs recommends looking at his family. This will help you understand what rules he was raised with in terms of how to handle loss and grief. Ask your husband, "How was it in your family when people died? What did you do about it?"

In some families death is never talked about. A person dies and is never mentioned again. If that's the background your husband comes from, then at least you'll be better able to understand that he's dealing with the miscarriage in a consistent way. That will help you understand he's not holding anything back from you, and that knowledge should help ease or at least allay some of the strain you're feeling over this issue.

But be sure to spend time working on whatever cracks the miscarriage caused in your marriage. As with your own emotional health, making sure that your marriage is healthy and on a proper track is important before you try to conceive again.

As the grief you felt over the loss of your pregnancy begins to ebb and your day-to-day life returns to normal, your thoughts will undoubtedly turn to having another baby. The next chapter will tell you everything you need to know in order to recognize when you are ready to try again.

6

▼

TRYING AGAIN

Getting to the point where you will be ready to conceive again involves two stages: physical healing and emotional healing. Most women find that their bodies heal sooner than their emotions. The important thing for you to do is to not put yourself under any pressure to conceive again. When you feel emotionally strong enough to start trying again—and strong enough to handle a subsequent loss, since losing a pregnancy is a risk everyone faces—then that's when you're ready.

There are other telltale signs to look for, too, and this chapter will tell you how to recognize when you're both physically and emotionally ready. It will detail what emotions you can expect to feel—or *not* to feel—during your subsequent pregnancy, how to make the decision as to whether you should tell people you are pregnant, and what to do should a loss occur again. It will also tell you when you should change doctors, when you should consult a specialist, and how to find one in your area.

DETERMINING WHEN YOU ARE PHYSICALLY READY

In order to give your uterus a chance to return to its normal size and your uterine lining a chance to rebuild itself, you should wait until you have two normal periods before you try conceiving again. You should get your first period four to eight weeks after the miscarriage, depending on how rapidly your HCG levels fall.

Although you will be able to have sex sooner, you should wait two weeks before resuming sexual intercourse so that your cervix has a chance to reclose, and so that you will, therefore, lessen your chance of infection.

....
When to Consult a Specialist

Anyone with any known diseases that may affect her pregnancy should have a consultation with either a high-risk pregnancy doctor, called a perinatalogist, or with a reproductive endocrinologist before even thinking about getting pregnant again. Your obstetrician will refer you to one of these specialists based on your illness.

If your doctor won't refer you to a specialist, you can find one yourself by looking up your diagnosis in a medical library and seeing where the most research on your condition is being done. Call that institution to get a referral in your geographic area. You may also contact the department of obstetrics and gynecology at a major academic institution in your area and ask the department chairman's office to give you a referral. Referrals can also be obtained from the American College of Obstetricians and Gynecologists, 409 12th Street, S.W., Washington D.C. 20024-2188, (202) 638-5577.

DECIDING WHEN YOU ARE EMOTIONALLY READY

Only you will be able to answer that question for yourself, but experts recommend giving yourself six months to recover emotionally before trying again. "Researchers have discovered that if parents conceive too soon after a loss, they may be unable to express their grief" over the miscarriage, thereby "delaying and complicating their emotional recovery," write Ingrid Kohn and Perry-Lynn Moffitt in *A Silent Sorrow*. "Grieving your baby is an absorbing process that may interfere with your ability to bond with your new child. If you fail to acknowledge and accept the loss before trying to have another child, you can fall into the trap of hoping to replace the baby you carried and lost."

Desperately wanting to conceive again is often a sign that "you may be wishing that the loss could be undone rather than feeling ready for another pregnancy," they write. "While the wish to replace the baby is understandable, it is important for you to mourn your loss before embarking on a new pregnancy."

"Obsessiveness about having another baby is often reflective of desperately trying to find a way of filling up your pain," says Sharon Covington. "You think that being pregnant is going to take your pain away. Thinking that way is dangerous because not only will your pain come back again at some point because it's not resolved, but you risk placing unrealistic expectations on your next child. Thinking that child will take away all your hurt and pain is a big burden to put on a little person."

So, be patient with yourself. Give yourself enough time to grieve your loss. You'll know when the intensity of your pain has eased and when any cracks in the foundation of your marriage, as discussed in the previous chapter, have been mended. Wait to conceive until you and your marriage are all right again, because then you will be able to love your next child for him or herself, and not as a baby to replace the one you lost or because of any expectations you have placed on him or her.

Also, to make sure you are not trying to replace the baby you lost, avoid giving the next baby the name you reserved for the baby you lost. If you do do that, you pass on all your hopes and dreams from one child to the next, and that's not fair to the subsequent child.

WHEN YOU'RE PREGNANT AGAIN

Once you've experienced miscarriage, you lose the ability to feel total joy in being pregnant. While most people know probems can occur in pregnancy, they tend to think those problems won't happen to them. You know firsthand those problems can indeed happen to you, and this knowledge may prevent you from bonding with the baby inside you the way you probably bonded with your first pregnancy. You're afraid to bond with the new pregnancy because you're afraid of losing this baby, too—afraid of feeling the kind of pain you felt over the first loss all over again. Some women are concerned about this failure to bond with their subsequent pregnancies, but this is a natural, self-protective mechanism and won't keep you from bonding with your baby once he or she is born.

Unfortunately, you probably won't enjoy your pregnancy the way you would have had you not lost the previous one. Early pregnancy, especially, will be an anxious time for you, but once you get past the due date of the pregnancy you lost, you'll find yourself feeling less anxious and, as the pregnancy progresses, you may even start to enjoy it.

WHEN TO TELL OTHERS ABOUT YOUR PREGNANCY

This decision is an extremely personal one. Only you will know what's right for you. If you didn't tell people you were pregnant before you miscarried, you may have felt compelled to keep your miscarriage a secret. This may have complicated your grieving process. On the other hand, you may have shared news of your pregnancy early on, only to then have to tell everyone—even the most casual of your acquaintances—that you miscarried. Perhaps when you lost that pregnancy you wished that you had kept quiet about it so that you would have been able to grieve in private.

Only you know how you felt after your miscarriage. Examine those feelings and think about what would have helped you be better able to deal with your feelings of grief. If you wanted your pregnancy to be recognized even though you lost it, then you may want to tell people about this pregnancy early on. You may also want to tell them about your miscarriage if you feel the need to have that loss be recognized. If you should lose this pregnancy, too, then you will have the emotional support you didn't have for the first one. Alternatively, if you wished for more privacy, then you may want to keep this pregnancy a secret until you are out of your first trimester. As with all personal decisions, simply do what feels right for you.

IF A LOSS OCCURS AGAIN

The most important step for you to take now is to undergo a physical evaluation for underlying problems that may be causing you to miscarry.

Emotionally, subsequent losses tend to be harder than the first. "Somehow you think that if you've been through an experience once it will be easier the next time around, but it's the opposite," says Covington. "It gets harder with each subsequent loss. There's a feeling that in some ways you're so near yet so far. You can conceive, yet you can't carry the pregnancy. It's like being duped, being fooled, which feels terribly humiliating in some ways for women. Women fear that they may never have a child or another child. Also, with each subsequent pregnancy that they lose they may begin to struggle with feelings that because something is wrong with them, they have killed their babies."

Most women find that the best thing for them to do to handle the emotions generated by repeat miscarriages—mainly fear that they will never have a baby and guilt that a medical condition that they have is taking their babies' lives—is to make sure they are getting the best possible medical care. They say this gives them a feeling of being at least a little in control of the situation, a feeling of knowing that they are doing something about it.

SHOULD YOU SWITCH DOCTORS?

Many women pick their obstetricians based on the recommendation of a friend or relative who used the doctor and liked her or him. Most women say they use their obstetrician because she or he is "nice."

Having a warm, empathetic doctor whom you feel comfortable with is wonderful, especially as you go through something as emotional as a pregnancy. However, just because your doctor is "nice" doesn't mean that she is the best doctor to be treating you, especially if you are repeatedly miscarrying. If an underlying physical condition is found to be causing your miscarriages, make sure you get the best medical care possible for your condition. Ask your doctor if she or he is qualified to treat your condition or if you would be better off in the hands of a specialist. If you have any doubts whatsoever about your doctor's ability to handle your condition, change doctors or seek out a specialist.

Of course, you should also change doctors if you think your obstetrician is not "nice." As with so many other personal decisions, only you can define what "nice" means to you. On the whole, you should feel comfortable talking to your doctor. She should be able to give you as much time as you need with her, and she should answer your questions clearly. If she doesn't, you should look elsewhere.

Many women who miscarry often feel that they are the only ones who have ever gone through the complicated grief and the sense of isolation that tend to follow a miscarriage. As you struggle with the emotions your miscarriage generated, it may be helpful to hear, in detail, the stories of other women's experiences with pregnancy loss.

In the following chapter, we hear from three different women as they tell us how their miscarriages affected them and their families. All three women have shared their stories in the hope that you—particularly if your miscarriage has left you feeling isolated from your friends and family—will know that you are not alone in your pain. They, too, suffered because of their miscarriages. They came through their suffering and, in time, so will you.

7

▼

THREE WOMEN'S STORIES

The first woman to tell her story miscarried once for an unknown reason. The story she tells of the shroud of silence she was expected to place over her grieving is one many women will be able to relate to.

The second woman suffered through six miscarriages, one ectopic pregnancy, and one stillbirth. Yet she never gave up hope that one day she would be able to carry to term. Her story illustrates how important it is to get proper medical care.

The third woman miscarried five times before she decided to adopt. And then she proved to herself, to her doctors, and to us that miracles do indeed sometimes happen.

IRENE DARIA
NUMBER OF MISCARRIAGES: ONE
CAUSE: UNKNOWN. ASSUMED TO BE A RANDOM
   CHROMOSOMAL ERROR

In early June 1993, my husband and I conceived our
first child. We conceived on our first try, and I was de-
lighted and amazed at how easy conception had
been. With infertility getting so much media cover-
age, I had wondered if I would have difficulty getting
pregnant even though nothing in my medical history
hinted at any such trouble. But many other dreams
in my life and in my husband Cary's life had been
achieved only after some struggle, and I'd thought
that having a baby, since it was so important to us,
might also involve some difficulty. Happily, it seemed
like it wouldn't. We began believing that in this one
area of our lives we'd been blessed.

Three weeks after my positive pregnancy test, I
had pain in my right ovary and was sent for a sonogram. I was afraid that the pain meant that something was wrong with the pregnancy, but I was told
that everything was fine. The pain was from a corpus
luteum cyst. The pregnancy was declared "viable."

I bonded with that unborn baby so quickly. Not
only had I been told that everything was fine, but I
had actually seen him (I thought of him as a boy from
the very beginning although, obviously, it was
too soon to know the baby's sex) on the black-and-
white sonogram monitor. He consisted of a yolk sac
within a gestational sac, and his shape was that of an
unshelled peanut. A white dot, the size of a pinpoint,

flickered in the yolk sac. That white dot was my baby's heart beating.

Seeing his heartbeat made my baby come alive for me. He became a person, even though he was only five weeks in the making (seven, if you count pregnancy weeks the way doctors do), even though he was hidden deep inside me, even though I could not yet feel him and there was not even the slightest bulge in my abdomen. From the moment I saw my baby, he began to take on an identity all his own.

Because of what he'd looked like on the screen, I nicknamed him Peanut, and Peanut became a part of my and Cary's daily life. It was summer and Cary tended to keep the air-conditioning on high. Over the next few weeks, whenever it got too cold I would say, "It's so cold in here that Peanut's put his ear-muffs on." Both of us would then imagine Peanut, snuggled up cozily inside me, wearing little red ear-muffs. When we gave our dog his little treats, we would give him three instead of his usual two. With the first treat we dropped into his waiting mouth, we'd say, "One from Mommy." The second treat: "One from Daddy." The third: "One from Peanut." Making Peanut a part of our daily routines added to our joy and kept the most amazing fact in the world never far from our minds—we were having a baby!

On Monday, July 19, 1993, our baby died. He went from being our much-wanted child to being a four-inch-wide clot of dark blood and dead tissue at the bottom of the toilet.

The symptoms of the miscarriage had started the previous Wednesday, although I didn't recognize them as such. That evening, while I was driving home from work I'd had a sharp, severe pain in my abdomen. It felt like the baby had huge jaws and was biting me.

Friday evening Cary and I went away for the weekend to Montauk, Long Island. That evening my sole pregnancy symptom—tender breasts—disappeared. Sunday afternoon I started having mild cramps. We went home and as the evening progressed, the cramps became slightly worse. I wasn't spotting and, although I was afraid that something might be wrong, I hoped that nothing was. After some time, I fell asleep.

At 2:00 A.M. I woke with a single terribly sharp pain in what I thought was my bladder. The mild menstrual cramps I'd been having had disappeared, and I took that as a sign of everything being all right with the pregnancy. I'd heard that cramps were what you had to worry about, and what I'd just felt wasn't a cramp. It was more like a stabbing pain, and I didn't think it had occurred anywhere near my uterus. Relieved that the cramps had disappeared, I went into the bathroom, urinated, and glanced down at the toilet paper without thinking much about what I was doing. I glanced at it the same way I'd glanced every time I'd gone to the bathroom since I'd learned I was pregnant, always to reassure myself that I wouldn't see what I saw now—a bright red streak of blood.

No!

I called my husband. He says he will never forget what my voice sounded like at that moment, the sadness contained in my single cry of "Cary!" Not fully awake, he stumbled into the bathroom. Wordlessly, I held out the toilet paper. He looked at the paper and then into the toilet and saw what I had not yet seen. When I looked into the toilet I couldn't believe that I hadn't felt such a large clump of blood fall out of me, and that it had made no sound as it slid into the toilet.

Both Cary and I handle emergencies well. Numb with shock, we did what we thought had to be done. Using a plastic container, he fished the bloody mass out of the toilet and placed it in the refrigerator. I left a message with my doctor's service. I had always thought that a miscarriage meant an emergency rush to the hospital, but the doctor on call said, "That's it. Go to Dr. Stevens'* office tomorrow morning, and he'll see if you've passed all of it or if you'll need a D&C to clean out any remaining dead tissue."

"That's it? There's nothing you can do?" I asked.

"That's it. I'm sorry."

Cary stretched out his arms. I walked into his embrace. Sensing that he expected me to cry, I did so but I stopped almost as quickly as I started. I didn't want to cry. What I wanted was an explanation. Why had this happened? My journalist's mind went into high gear, searching for answers.

A woman I knew who lived near Montauk had suffered two miscarriages. I'd heard of another woman who had been vacationing in Montauk when she miscarried. Was there some connection between my miscarrying and my having just been in Montauk? Women on Long Island have a high rate of breast cancer, and I wondered if they had a high rate of mis-

*The name of my doctor has been changed.

carriage, too. I wondered if some kind of environmental pollutants on Long Island could have caused my miscarriage. Wanting answers, I asked my husband to access Nexis on our computer and research the answers to my questions for me.

It was three o'clock in the morning. We had just lost a baby. We weren't crying. We weren't holding each other. We weren't talking. The only sound in the room was the click of computer keys as my husband tried to find the answer to the only thing I could think at that moment, Why?

We found no answers. Fifteen minutes later, my husband stopped typing and gently said, "This is ridiculous."

I'd been reading the computer screen over his shoulder and as we were finding no answers to my questions, as I was deciding my questions were unanswerable and probably of no merit, the fact that we'd lost our baby had begun to sink in. This wasn't someone else's life that I was researching. This wasn't a story I was about to write. This was my life. The life that had just ended was my baby's. By the time my husband deemed our endeavor ridiculous, I had come to the same conclusion.

Cary and I sat on the couch and held each other. I cried, but my tears were strange ones. Automatic ones. They weren't really an expression of sadness. They were more a release of the tension caused by shock and by a strong feeling of disbelief. When I'd gone to sleep I'd been pregnant, and now I wasn't. How could things have changed so fast, so unexpectedly?

Every twenty minutes or so I urinated and passed more blood clots. Although these clots were much smaller than the first, I could feel them as they came out of me. Passing those clots involved no physical pain—not even cramps—but the emotional pain caused by knowing that those clots contained minuscule pieces of my baby was too enormous to process and to feel. My tears continued to fall, but inside I was numb.

The next morning, when we told my in-laws I had miscarried, my mother-in-law cried, "Oh! I'm so glad I didn't tell any of my friends that you were pregnant."

That was my first inkling of the way miscarriage is handled. It is cloaked in silence. My mother-in-law was clearly implying that something unmentionable had happened to me. Her words made me feel ashamed of the fact that I had miscarried. Her words made me feel relieved that so few people had known of my pregnancy. Only my family and my two closest friends had been aware of it. No one at work had known and now no one—except for my boss, who I felt deserved to know the truth behind why I would be calling in sick—would ever know. No one would know because, without even thinking about why I was doing it, I had followed our society's unwritten law—that of not announcing your pregnancy until you're safely out of your first trimester. Of course, I understood that this secrecy existed just in case something should go wrong. But I never followed this reasoning to its logical conclusion, which, of course, is that if you did lose your baby no one would know about your loss. I was about to find out that the fact that few people know of your loss complicates and extends your grieving immeasurably.

That same morning I called my obstetrician's office and was told to come in right away. I had never met Dr. Stevens before. My previous gynecologist didn't deliver babies. Dr. Stevens had delivered a friend's baby. She'd raved about him and, trusting her opinion, I'd picked him as my obstetrician sight unseen. As a rule, Dr. Stevens doesn't examine patients who are pregnant for the first time until they are eight weeks into the pregnancy. I was scheduled to have my first appointment with him in two days.

Luckily, he was a nice guy. He said how sorry he was that we were meeting under these circumstances, and I began to cry again. He handed me a box of tissues and, trying to make me feel better, he said, "Miscarriage is very common. It's no big deal. You'll go on to have healthy babies. In a few months you'll try again. My mother had three healthy children and two miscarriages. It happens to everyone."

"Everyone?"

"One out of four women."

"If that's true then why don't I know more women who had miscarried?"

"Because that's the way miscarriage is handled. People don't talk about it."

Cary and I must have looked skeptical because Dr. Stevens continued, "You'll see. If you decide to tell your friends what happened you'll be amazed at the number who'll say, 'I had a miscarriage, too.' And if not them, their relatives or best friends will have had one."

We wanted to believe him, wanted to think that what had happened to us was indeed common and that most people did go on to have healthy babies after their miscarriages. We exchanged a look, my husband shrugged, and we both filed that information away in our minds as something to be examined later.

At that moment we had more urgent things to take care of. My husband held up the opaque plastic container containing the pregnancy specimen. "We saved this," he said. Although the doctor couldn't see into the container he clearly knew what was inside.

He shook his head no. "It's not worth sending out for testing. The lab won't be able to tell anything from it." He didn't tell us why, although I now know it's because the water in the toilet bowl had killed the live pregnancy cells needed for genetic testing. Dr. Stevens said we should assume that what had gone wrong was a random chromosomal error.

We said we didn't want to just assume what had gone wrong. We wanted a definite answer. But the doctor remained firm. A test that would tell us the reason for this miscarriage could not be performed, and, without fully understanding why that was the case, we finally accepted what he said.

He sent me for a sonogram, which confirmed the pregnancy was no longer viable but showed that some residual tissue still remained inside my uterus. Like Dr. Stevens, the radiologist who performed the sonogram told us that miscarriage was more common than we thought. "It's so common that doctors don't even do any diagnostic testing, don't even go looking for possible sources of trouble until a woman has had two consecutive miscarriages," she said. "You'll see," she added, "it happens to everyone."

She called Dr. Stevens to confirm that it had happened to me. We talked to him on the phone from the radiologist's office. He told us to go to the hospital, and he would perform the D&C at 5:00 P.M. Still wanting an answer, we asked if anything he retrieved during the D&C could be sent for chromosomal analysis, and he said he doubted it. Then, sounding like he was just placating us, he said, "But I'll see what I find during the procedure."

I spent the rest of the day lying in a hospital bed with Cary sitting on its edge and holding my hand. Neither one of us cried. We were still in shock. Were we really here? Was it really just yesterday that we were on the beach, me reading *What to Expect When You're Expecting*? We certainly hadn't expected this.

At around five o'clock, an orderly wheeled me to the operating room. Even the ride on the gurney felt surreal. It was so smooth that it seemed as if the halls of the hospital were moving and I was stationary. As I was wheeled by people in the halls, everyone stopped talking and stared at me. *Everyone* stared—doctors, nurses, orderlies, visitors, patients walking the halls strapped to their IVs. My usual spunkiness reappeared briefly, and I stared right back at them. My stare had its intended effect—they looked away.

Getting those people to stop staring at me was important to me because it was the only thing I could control. Everything else had spun out of control. I'd lost a baby, and now I was being wheeled to an operating room to have a surgical procedure that would be performed by a doctor I'd met for the first time earlier that day. I was scared.

After the anesthesia had been hooked up, Dr. Stevens strode into the room, dressed in his surgical scrubs. "Hello," he said, as chipper as if we were running into each other at a cocktail party. "How are you?"

His lighthearted tone sent a clear signal that he didn't want to hear the truth. I was terrified, but I didn't say that. This man was about to do a surgical procedure on me. I wasn't about to ruffle his feathers. I would take my cues from him, and so I said, "Fine." And then I watched and listened in disbelief as—while I lay on the operating table needing consolation, support, and empathy—Dr. Stevens started telling the head anesthesiologist all about the vacation he'd just returned from in France. I wanted to know exactly how he was going to get this dead tissue out from inside of me and what the procedure would feel like. Instead, I learned that he and his wife had hired a driver and spent the past two weeks touring the French countryside.

This doctor might have excellent technical skills, as I'd been told, but Marcus Welby he wasn't. Giving him the benefit of the doubt, I decided that maybe he needed to keep an emotional distance from a patient he was about to do an invasive procedure on. But I had needs, too. Politely, I interrupted his travelogue and asked him what he was about to do to me.

Immediately, he came over and said that a screen would be placed across my chest so that I wouldn't be able to see anything he was doing. He said he would then dilate my uterus and scrape out the contents and . . .

The next thing I remember is waking up in the recovery room. Dr. Stevens was there. Having recovered his ability to empathize, he asked how I was feeling, and he seemed to want a genuine answer. I was fine, just sleepy. He said everything had gone perfectly, and that I would be going back to my room soon. He said he'd found nothing that could be sent for genetic testing, and, again, he said that we should assume that what went wrong was a fluke, a random chromosomal error. He asked if my husband was in my room. I said yes, and he went to tell my husband that I was fine.

Physically, I *was* fine. Emotionally, things were another story. The eight weeks after the miscarriage remain the most confusing, fuzzy, foggy time of my entire life. I was mourning the loss of a baby that had never been fully created, a baby I had never met. I was mourning, but very few people knew that. Therefore, almost everyone I came in contact with expected me to be my usual chipper self, and I tried to accommodate them.

I put up a good façade. No one at work could tell how much I was hurting, even though for two whole weeks I cried as I drove to work. I cried at lunchtime as I sat in my car in the park near my office. I cried on my way home from work. But I never cried at work, not even when three of my co-workers, one by one, announced that they were pregnant. I showed no outward sign of how each of their announcements sent a slice of pain and jealousy right through me.

Since none of my pregnant co-workers knew of my miscarriage, none of them saw any reason to temper their joy over their impending motherhood to accommodate my grief. One of these pregnant women posted on her department's bulletin board a large sketch of her baby's current stage of in-utero development—a stage my own baby would soon have been approaching—even though this bulletin board was in my immediate line of sight. Every time I looked up from my word processor, I had to stare at a diagram of what my baby would have looked like, had he lived. When this same woman raised her shirt in the office kitchen to show off her pregnant belly, she didn't lower her shirt when I walked in, not knowing that I wouldn't want to see what my own belly would soon have looked like, too. Everywhere I turned in the office there was talk of babies.

Illogically and unfairly, I was upset with my co-workers because none of them had expressed condolences over my miscarriage. But how could they express condolences over a loss they knew nothing about? But my loss was so great, so life-altering, that I was surprised there was no visible manifestation of it the way there would be if you lost a limb. I had lost an important part of myself. I had lost a child, lost my hopes and dreams for this baby. I was fundamentally changed, yet everyone treated me exactly the way they had before and expected me to act the way I had before—to chitchat and to joke and to laugh in between the time we spent getting our jobs done. Like a young woman who's just lost her virginity and looks at herself in the mirror and is surprised that she doesn't look different, I looked at the lighthearted way my co-workers treated me and thought to myself, "Can't they tell what's just happened to me? Can't they see?"

Just as I didn't cry at work, I rarely cried at home. Cary said he wanted to put the miscarriage behind him and focus on the future instead of on the past. Unless I raised the subject, he never talked about it, and when I did raise the subject he got annoyed. This was so not like my always-willing-to-listen husband that I should have realized he was struggling with his own grief in his own way. Instead, I thought he really had put the miscarriage behind him. His ability to do it so quickly made me feel like the overwhelming grief I was just beginning to feel was inappropriate.

My two best friends and my parents and in-laws made me feel that way, too. After the first week, none of them ever brought up the miscarriage again. But I would bring it up, and when I told them I was feeling sad, many of them asked if I wanted to go talk to "someone" about it. I had to be asked that question a few times before I stopped replying, "I am talking to someone about it. I'm talking to you." Finally, I realized that, by "someone" they meant a therapist.

My friends and family wanted me to return to being my usual cheerful, resilient self. Trying to speed that process along, they would say things they thought would be consoling, things like, "At least you know you're fertile" or "You'll have another baby." What I really needed to hear one of them say was, "I can understand why you're feeling so sad." But not one of them said that. I started keeping my sadness to myself and began to feel more and more isolated from everyone I loved. They stopped calling me, and I stopped calling them. I couldn't control what I was feeling, and I didn't want to talk to people who made me feel like what I was feeling was inappropriate.

Even remembering what my doctor had said on the day of the miscarriage made me feel like my grief was inappropriate. He'd meant well when he down-played the significance of my miscarriage. But I wish he'd made it sound a little more significant, because about a week after the miscarriage, when the shock had worn off and I was ready to begin grieving, his words returned to haunt me: "It's no big deal. . . . It happens to everyone. . . . In a few months you'll try again." If it was no big deal, why was I carrying around such a bottomless well of sadness? Why did I feel as if life would never be the same, as if I would never again find pleasure in anything?

I tried to bury my grief, tried to be more like my husband and forget about it. But I couldn't. The more I tried to ignore my grief, the more depressed I got. And the more depressed I got, the more I couldn't understand why I was so depressed. Now it seems clear. I'd lost a baby. I'd lost the closeness I'd always felt with my husband, the connection I'd felt with my friends, and the bond I'd felt with my family. Never, ever, had I felt so isolated.

I also began feeling an odd sense of shame. Intellectually, I certainly wasn't ashamed about my miscarriage. But because of the secrecy that surrounded it I began to feel like I'd experienced something shameful, and that was a terrible feeling.

I reached rock bottom five weeks after the miscarriage when Cary left for a two-week business trip to South America. With him gone I had no reason, and no way, to ignore my grief or distract myself from it. I have never felt such sadness in my whole life. I needed help dealing with this level of grief, and with my friends and family having shown themselves incapable of giving me the kind of support I needed, I turned to a place I was sure would be able to help me through this—the huge neighborhood bookstore.

Since my doctor had said that miscarriage was such an everyday occurrence in pregnancies, I expected to find a plethora of books on the subject in the pregnancy section. To my surprise, there was only one book, and that was on how to prevent miscarriages. That certainly wasn't going to do me any good. A salesclerk directed me to the death and dying section where I found only one book that dealt with the emotional aspects of miscarriage and stillbirth. The title of that book, interestingly enough, was *Silent Sorrow*.

At first I was appalled at the fact that this book on something I was trying to think of as a natural part of the pregnancy process had been placed in the death and dying section. As it turned out, seeing where that book was placed was the best thing that could have happened. It was the beginning of the validation of why I was feeling so horrible—I had experienced the death of a baby. An unborn baby but, still, a baby.

Reading the book helped a lot. The book made me realize it really was fine to feel so sad. The book said that people who had never experienced miscarriage would try to discount your grief, which made me feel less angry at, and disappointed in, the people I loved. The book made me realize that other women had experienced exactly what I was going through—the terrible feeling of being so isolated within your sadness. The book also made me realize that I had to start talking to Cary about how I was feeling.

He called that night from South America, as he'd called every night. I'd been saying I was fine, but that night I told him how upset I really was and how hard a time I was having dealing with the miscarriage all alone. He got on a plane that night and flew home, he thought, to support me. We ended up supporting each other.

Cary read *Silent Sorrow*, too, and it unlocked his own grief. He said he'd been depressed but had been throwing himself into work, not sure why he was feeling so bad but not wanting to examine it. He, too, had been replaying the doctor's words in his mind and hadn't known why he was feeling so terrible about something the doctor had said was "no big deal." Cary and I are two intelligent people who are in touch with our feelings, so it's amazing that we needed a book to tell us it was all right to grieve. But we did.

We spent the next week at home together, reconnecting and talking about our loss. Then, feeling much better, we faced the world again. This time, supported by what we'd read and by each other, we felt our grief was normal, and as we began to feel that way we both found that we needed to tell people outside our innermost circle about the miscarriage.

What Dr. Stevens had predicted came to pass. We were shocked at how many of our acquaintances—a full 75 percent of them—had suffered through a miscarriage, too. Silently. Why hadn't they told us about their miscarriages? We wondered, but we didn't ask. It didn't seem important. What *was* important was that we knew about their miscarriages now. That knowledge made us realize that miscarriage really was a common occurrence and that we shouldn't be too worried about it, which we had been. All of these people who had miscarriages now had children. That fact gave us both great consolation.

All of those people had also been surprised by how many of their friends and acquaintances and sometimes even their family members had not told them about their own miscarriages. One woman never knew her mother had experienced a miscarriage until she miscarried herself. It was while consoling her that her mother let her secret slip.

My own secret slipped at work for the same reason—I reached out to console a co-worker who miscarried a baby shortly after I did. She miscarried quite late in her pregnancy, so there was no way for her to keep it a secret. I called her at home and said, "I just want you to know how sorry I am for you and that I know how you feel. I had a miscarriage, too." The moment I said those words, relief flooded through me. My sense of shame, my sense that I had something terrible to hide from the general public began to disappear. It was freeing to have my secret be out in my office.

My secret was out and so were the secrets of others. On my way to the door that night I passed two women sitting at their desks. One said, "I had some spotting and cramping." The other replied, "That's what happened to me, too." Immediately, I knew what they were talking about, and, not caring who else heard, I stopped and said, "I had a miscarriage, too."

Those two women and I talked about how isolated we'd felt after our miscarriages and how people who had never had miscarriages themselves became strangely uncomfortable if we raised the subject. We talked about how not the grief but the inability to talk openly about our grief had nearly destroyed us. We talked about how silence had been expected of us, and I told them how the only book I had been able to find in the bookstore on the emotional reaction to miscarriage had been called *Silent Sorrow.*

The three of us at work certainly were silent no more. We all went home that night feeling good. In fact, one of the women felt so good about our conversation that, that night, she told a female friend of hers about it, a friend who had never known about her miscarriage. What did her friend say in response? Words that I now expect to hear, more often than not, when I tell someone about my own miscarriage. Her friend said, "I had a miscarriage, too."

I became pregnant again in January of 1994. Throughout the pregnancy I checked for blood every time I urinated. Every abdominal cramp I felt (and you feel a lot of them when you're pregnant) made me stop what I was doing to analyze the type of cramp. Because I knew things could go wrong all the way up to the time of delivery, I was guarded in my happiness, in a way I had not been guarded during my first pregnancy.

Even though I was guarded in my joy, I announced my pregnancy right away. Not only did my family members and friends know I was pregnant, but so did my co-workers, my neighbors, and even the owners of the dogs our dog plays with in the park. I told them all—even the most casual of these acquaintances—about my miscarriage too. Just as I needed my new pregnancy to be recognized, I needed the loss of my previous pregnancy to be recognized as well. I no longer felt ashamed about the miscarriage, and I needed people to accept my miscarriage as a fact of my life. I also needed to know that if I miscarried my new pregnancy, too, I would be allowed to mourn openly and purely, with no sense of secrecy or shame complicating an already complicated process.

Thankfully, nothing went wrong. I delivered seven-pound, fourteen-ounce Jameson Grant on October 6, 1994. At the time of this writing he's twelve months old, and he's an absolute delight. Since I was so afraid to bond with him during my pregnancy for fear that I would lose him, too, I was afraid to ever imagine him as an actual baby. I always thought of him as my pregnancy. Therefore, it took me about seven months after he was born to fully absorb the fact that I was actually a mother and that he was actually my baby. But I've absorbed it.

I never thought I would ever be writing or thinking or saying these words, but I rarely think about my miscarriage anymore. Jamie has a lot to do with that. People say you never forget your miscarriage, and that's certainly true. They say it changes you forever, and that's true, too. But it changed me and my husband and my marriage for the better. The miscarriage initially pushed us apart, but once we finally talked about what we were feeling, it brought us closer together. And, indirectly, the miscarriage brought us Jamie. On the one hand, I wish I hadn't miscarried, yet at the same time I wouldn't trade Jamie for any other baby in the world. The miscarriage has become a sad part of my past that no longer colors my present. I couldn't ask for a better resolution.

KAREN HESS
NUMBER OF MISCARRIAGES: SIX, PLUS ONE STILLBIRTH
    AND ONE ECTOPIC PREGNANCY
CAUSE: ANTIPHOSPHOLIPID SYNDROME

The main thing I learned after losing eight pregnancies and then, finally, carrying a healthy baby to term is this: If you know you have a problem, go out and find yourself a doctor who is associated with a university hospital. This is especially true if it's a newly recognized problem like my antiphospholipid syndrome was when I was trying to have a baby. There's so much research going on at universities that the doctors who work at those hospitals are usually up on the latest research, and if they aren't, they can confer with the doctors around them who are.

Don't do what I did, which was go to obstetricians my friends and family members referred me to. Most people think that if their obstetrician is nice then he or she will be able to help you. They give you that reference, and when you're desperate you'll listen to anything. I learned the hard way that just because someone's nice doesn't necessarily mean they know enough to help you. You have to be candid with the doctor and ask point blank, "Are you qualified to handle this problem, and if you're not would you kindly refer me to someone who is?"

The really good doctors will recognize when they can't do something and will refer you to a specialist. But sometimes doctors think they can handle something that they simply cannot. I don't blame my doctors for my losses, but I do think that if I'd gone to the group of doctors who saw me through my last, successful pregnancy sooner, I would have lost fewer pregnancies.

I began the long, slow process of learning this in 1985 when, at the age of 32, I miscarried my first pregnancy at eight weeks. My husband and I hadn't told anyone about the pregnancy. If something went wrong and I had a miscarriage, I wanted us to deal with it privately, which is what we did. John and I didn't even tell our families.

I lost the pregnancy naturally. There wasn't any kind of procedure or anything involved. It was upsetting, of course, but we didn't make much of the loss. The doctor told me that one in three pregnancies ends up in miscarriage or in some other problem. I knew miscarriage was common. I figured that, like the doctor said, these things happen. It's a normal part of pregnancy, and we would just try again.

The second miscarriage was in 1987. Again, I went to eight weeks and started bleeding and cramping. With that one I had to have a D&C. I had to take some time off from work, and so I had to tell some people about what had happened. I found that it helped to talk about it because I found out that just about every woman I knew had either had a miscarriage or had a friend or family member who had one. I was amazed that there were so many miscarriages going on around me that I didn't know about because people just don't talk about it. Knowing that made me feel better because I was still trying to think that my own miscarriages were like most other women's—a normal fact of life—and that I didn't have any underlying problem.

My mind wanted to believe that, but in my heart I began to feel I might have a problem. My own doctor was convinced that I didn't, and he wouldn't run any tests until I'd had another miscarriage, so when a friend of mine suggested I go and see her doctor, I went. Like my previous doctor, this one also said that most likely there wasn't anything to be concerned about, but that he would do a physical workup on me to see if everything was okay. He did all the standard tests, like checking my uterus and tubes with a hysterosalpingogram and sending both my husband and me for a genetic workup. Everything came back normal.

Encouraged by that, I conceived again in 1989. At first, remembering my initial two losses, I was guarded and wouldn't let myself be happy. But everything progressed normally. I passed the eight week point where I'd lost the previous pregnancies, and I didn't lose this one. I had amniocentesis done at 15 weeks, and John and I spent the next four weeks worrying that something was going to come back out of the ordinary. At 19 weeks we got the phone call saying the baby was a healthy boy. John and I finally let ourselves be happy and, God, were we elated.

The next week I felt a sharp pain in my abdomen and saw a few drops of blood. I was terrified that I was losing the baby. I went to my doctor's office. My doctor wasn't in, so I saw his associate. I lay down on the examining table, and he put the Doppler monitor on my stomach to hear the baby's heartbeat and there was . . . silence.

Callously, the doctor blurted out, "Your baby's dead."

Even now, six years later, I can't talk about the loss of that baby without crying. That was the worst thing that ever happened to me. I don't think I could ever feel that pain again. That loss was harder than the first two miscarriages because the pregnancy had gone so far. I knew he was a boy. I knew he was healthy. I'd heard his heartbeat. I'd felt him moving. To know and experience all that and then to be told, "Your baby's dead," was very, very difficult.

I never said anything to my doctor's associate about

how brutally he had told me the news. All I said was that I didn't want the associate to induce labor in me when I went into the hospital. I said I wanted my regular doctor to do the procedure, and he did.

Before the doctor induced labor he asked if I wanted to see or hold the baby. I said no. There are certain things I can and can't do, and looking at that baby was one thing I knew I could never do. I would have remembered that sight for the rest of my life.

The doctor recommended that I not have a funeral for the baby. He said they would handle the disposal of it. Sometimes I question whether I should have had a funeral to put a closure on the loss, but I think for me it would have been worse to have a gravesite today. I often wonder whether they used the fetus for research and if he did any good for anybody, but I don't dwell on it. I'm settled with the decision I made at the time.

A lot of people had known I was pregnant. After the stillbirth, I asked several people to spread the word that I had had a problem, and I asked people not to talk to me about it because I was afraid I wouldn't have been able to hold it together during any conversation on the subject.

It was a very difficult time. I was so sad. *So* depressed. I took a year and a half leave of absence from work to try and get over losing the baby. The previous losses had hurt, but they hadn't hurt as much as the stillbirth. To me the first two pregnancies weren't real babies. At eight weeks they were pregnancies. The pain and the mourning that I went through for that year and a half was just for the loss of that one baby, that boy. That baby was always in my mind.

It was a very difficult time, and John and I helped each other get through it. We didn't talk to any other people about how sad we were feeling. Before the loss of that baby, I'd never looked at my husband as being vulnerable at all. Most times he's very, very strong. For the first time I saw him in pain. He'd lost a baby, too. Dealing with the loss together brought us closer. I realized I was married to a real nice man, someone I really cared for and who really cared for me, which is not what I could say about my doctor, at least not at that time.

My doctor was going through his own personal crisis, dealing with his wife's serious illness, and his mind wasn't completely focused on his work. When I went back for my follow-up appointment two weeks later, it was one, two, three, and I was out the door. He told me the autopsy on the baby had revealed that the cause of death had been "insufficient placenta." That's what happens when you have my condition—the blood vessels in the placenta get all clogged so that the baby doesn't get enough oxygen or nutrients. But no one knew I had this condition yet, so at the time they couldn't give me a reason as to why the placenta hadn't developed properly.

This doctor said the same words my previous doctor had said about my miscarriages: "It was just one of those things."

I left his office thinking, "Okay, it was one of those things." But in my heart I knew it couldn't possibly be just one of those things. I started blaming myself for the loss. I thought, "All my tests came back normal. There's no physical reason for me to be losing these babies. I must be doing something wrong." Because of the nature of my job, I do a lot of walking around. I thought maybe I should have quit working. I knew it couldn't possibly be happening so many times without there being a reason, but I couldn't imagine what that reason was.

My depression over the loss of that baby started to lift once I got past the baby's due date. That summer of 1990, another friend of mine suggested another doctor she'd heard was very good, and I went to see him. He was surprised that my previous doctor hadn't done an immunological workup. He explained to me that there could be something called anticardiolipin antibodies causing my problem. He had me go for the test and it turned out that I was producing these anticardiolipin antibodies, and they were causing the blood clots in my placenta.

The best thing I ever heard was to be told that the doctor knew the cause of the problem. I was so relieved and thrilled to know it wasn't something I had done or didn't do, and also no one would ever say to me again, "Oh, it's just one of those things." There was a problem, and that meant there might be a treatment for it. At that time, in 1990, doctors knew of the problem, but the method of treatment for it was very much trial and error.

This doctor waited until I got pregnant again, and when I did he put me on aspirin to thin my blood and on prednisone, a steroid that suppresses the immune system and causes horrible side effects. When I

say horrible, I mean *horrible*. I was on a large dose—
40 mgs a day—and it caused my whole body and my
whole personality to change. First, my face swelled
up like a big balloon. All of my features got distorted.
I got huge black-and-blue marks and mouth sores. I
was getting infections in my mouth because the prednisone suppressed my immune system.

Even worse, my whole attitude about life changed.
I just couldn't have cared less. I'd think, "If I get hit
by a truck, so what?" You don't view life the same way
when you're on that drug. They give prednisone to
dogs for allergies. When I know a dog is on prednisone, I stay away from the dog because I know what
I was like when I was on prednisone. You have a *bad*
attitude.

I hated being on prednisone, but I figured I'd only
have to endure this for nine months and it would all
be worth it if I could have a baby. But the pregnancy
wasn't right from the beginning. I was having a heavy
discharge of blood, my HCG count was never right,
and the doctor kept checking me sonographically
and saying he didn't see anything in the uterus. He
started checking me at five weeks and he said, "I have
bad news. I'm convinced you're either miscarrying
or you have an ectopic pregnancy." But he waited another three weeks before my HCG count and my
sonogram findings absolutely convinced him that it
was ectopic. He said I would have to have immediate
surgery to remove my right fallopian tube. So, in
December 1990, I had my right tube removed.

The doctor said that the ectopic pregnancy had
nothing to do with my condition. He said, "Don't

worry, Karen, you can always try again." What went through my mind was *"Forget it. You're out of your mind. This is nuts."* I was very emotional. I kept thinking, "I just don't get this. It doesn't make sense to me. My diagnosis was supposed to be the answer for everything, and now I've lost another pregnancy."

This doctor may have been a good physician, but his bedside manner was abominable. When I went in for the surgery he told my husband, "This will take only fifteen minutes, and we'll be out. Everything will be fine." Well, two and a half hours later after we came out of the operating room, he only gave my husband a minute. He said, "Everything's fine." John wanted to talk to him, but he had to hurry on his way.

Maybe if that doctor's bedside manner had been different we would have tried again, but at that point John said, "Karen, enough of this nonsense. Let's stop this. Don't ever go back to that guy. Let's start looking into other options."

John wanted to adopt a baby, but I wasn't interested. I was scared to. I had family members offer to carry a baby for me. There were lots of options open to me, but I never considered any of them. I wanted to carry our baby, and if I couldn't do that then I didn't want to have children at all.

I was still on my leave of absence, but I decided to go back to work. I thought, "That's all I'm going to do for the rest of my life—work. I don't want to be a parent anymore. I don't want any of this anymore. It's over with." And my husband agreed.

Ten months went by. We had just resigned ourselves to the idea of not having children when a cousin of mine said that a friend of hers who had had problems carrying to term had gone to a doctor who was very good. My cousin suggested that I give him a shot. My husband didn't want me to go. He said, "Do you really want to go through this again?"

I had become very knowledgeable about pregnancy loss by then. I knew that the ectopic pregnancy really had been just a fluke that had nothing to do with my condition, so I went to this doctor.

He did his own testing and confirmed my previous diagnosis. But he said I shouldn't have been put on prednisone after I'd gotten pregnant. I should have been on it *before* I'd gotten pregnant. But treatment really was still trial and error. I could tell that because he said to me, "How much prednisone did the other doctor have you on?" and when I told him he said, "Oh well, maybe we'll increase it." I could tell he really didn't know exactly what he was doing. The approach seemed to be, "Okay that didn't work so let's try a little bit more."

He recommended my taking prednisone and aspirin for two months before conceiving. I was beside myself having to go on prednisone again, because I knew what awful things were going to happen to me. I didn't want to take the prednisone again, but then I thought, "Well, this is the second doctor who uses this method of treatment, so this is probably what I should be doing. And it's not going to be forever. It's just nine months."

He put me on 60 mgs of prednisone a day. That's a very high dose, and one night it made my heart race. I called the doctor. He was away, and when his part-

ner found out the amount I was on, he was flabber-
gasted and told me, "I think you'd better cut down
immediately."

I did and I conceived again and had another miscarriage at about six or eight weeks. That was devastating. To go through all that torture with the
prednisone and think that maybe this was going to
be the answer and then to lose the pregnancy . . .

The doctor just shook his head and said, "You really should stop doing this. You should adopt." He
wrote me off. He didn't want to be bothered. I had
told him my history, and he knew I was doing my own
research and that I was doctor hopping. I think he
got nervous when he saw me trying to take matters
into my own hands. He didn't like that, and he didn't
want anything more to do with me. He'd tried what
he thought was best according to what he'd read
about my condition and it didn't work, so that was
that. I think he was doing this on a wing and a prayer.

To a lot of these doctors you're just a folder. You're
a file. I just kind of took it as a matter of course that
doctors are cold or seem to hold back information. I
always came out of their offices thinking, "Do they
know what they're talking about, or is it that they
think I won't understand what they're talking about?"
They could never really explain things to me; they
would never get involved in talking to me. I always
came out shaking my head thinking, "Am I doing the
right thing?" But of course you're hopeful and you
think, "I'll give it one more shot. How bad could it
be? I could go through one more operation if that's
the worse thing that happens."

At this point one side of me was saying, "You'll never try it again," and then the other side would say, "Yes you will. You're still young. You'll find a way to treat this, and it will be fine." But for the most part I was going about my day to day business thinking, "Well, we'll never have a family."

After losing that last pregnancy in January 1992, I stopped going to doctors. Every once in a while I would say to John, "Gee I'm sorry I can't give you a baby," and he would say, "I didn't marry you for your breeding capabilities." But I always felt very bad. When you're the one causing the problem, you're very hard on yourself. John and I would never dwell on it, but there would be days when I would sit there and feel very bad because I knew John would make a great father.

I wasn't trying to get pregnant; I wasn't on any treatment for my condition. My next three pregnancies were accidents. They happened six months apart, and all were unsuccessful. I was using spermicide as my method of birth control. (Because of my condition I can't use the Pill because it increases your risk of blood clots, and I don't like the diaphragm.) I wasn't as careful as I should have been. I guess subconsciously I thought maybe there was a chance. I never really gave up hope completely.

When I got pregnant with the first of those last three pregnancies, I went back to my second doctor, the one who had been having a personal crisis when I'd last seen him. I went back to that doctor because I wasn't actively looking to have kids anymore, and he was a nice man. I was almost embarrassed to call him each time. I kept thinking, "I've got to do something to get this birth control under control."

All the doctor kept saying was, "I'm sorry." He never did say, "Do you want to try having a baby? Do you want to see a specialist?" I didn't know how much research was being done on my condition. I didn't know that there were doctors out there who were highly qualified to treat women with antiphospholipid syndrome.

With those three pregnancies I never even got off the running board. I have very regular menstrual cycles. I'm 27 or 28 days on the button with getting my period. If I went for 31 days I would know I was pregnant. I would take the home pregnancy test, go to the doctor, and confirm I was pregnant. Each time, he'd say my HCG levels didn't look good and to prepare myself for another loss. Each time, I'd start bleeding within a week.

Every miscarriage hurts. You can be pregnant for just two days, and it still hurts when you lose it. I didn't want to go through that hurt anymore, and I started thinking about having my remaining tube tied, but I didn't. Although intellectually I was saying that I wasn't going to try again, something inside kept saying . . . maybe.

In March of 1993 I started having some neurological problems. I started forgetting a lot of things. At first I thought I was being inattentive, but then it got worse. I started not completing tasks. I would set the coffee pot up, put water in, and never put the coffee in. I'd get the washing machine going and forget to put the clothes in. I made excuses. I thought I was overworked. Then I started having real problems with numbers. If someone gave me a phone number to write down, I couldn't do it. I'd transpose the numbers. That really concerned me because part of my business was numbers. Then just being able to communicate became difficult. Sometimes I couldn't find the words that I wanted. I had to struggle sometimes just to complete a thought. It was a daily problem, and it was getting worse. It got so I wouldn't want to talk to someone because I knew I wouldn't be able to say what I wanted to say. Now I know what people with Alzheimer's and dementia go through. It's a frightening thing when you're losing your mind. Of course, I didn't want to think that there could be a physical problem. I just wanted to think I just had to get my act together.

All along, I'd say to my husband, "Strange things are happening," and he'd say, "Karen, you're just preoccupied. You have to start doing one thing at a time." I wanted to believe him, but I knew there was something wrong. I was really afraid to go to the doctor because I was afraid he'd find something really serious. I should have gone to the doctor, but I didn't.

Then one day my husband said, "Karen, you're acting so weird. What's with you? Knock it off."

I don't remember what I'd done that caused him to say that but I do remember thinking, "Oh God. I can't hide this anymore. Now it's not just me that's recognizing it. Other people are recognizing it. I'd better do something about this."

That was in August. I didn't want to go to the doctor again and so I thought, "Well, you hear so much about aspirin being the cure-all for everything, I'm going to start taking an aspirin every day." After two weeks of taking a low-dose baby aspirin every day, all of my symptoms cleared up. In October I got pregnant by accident again. I didn't even call the doctor because I was waiting to lose the pregnancy, but I didn't. I said, "Oooh, maybe this aspirin is working."

With every other pregnancy, although I missed my period, I would have some slight spotting right from the start. With this one I didn't have any in the beginning. That was the first time that had happened to me. I put off taking the home pregnancy test because I just didn't want to start the whole thing all over again. I thought, "Oh God, if I'm pregnant how will it end this time? Is it going to be ectopic in the other tube? Will I need a D&C this time? How long am I going to have to wait to lose it?" I didn't want to deal with any of those questions, so I kept putting off taking the test. I kept thinking, "It'll come, it'll come" because I felt crampy and bloated and thought, "I'm getting older, and maybe I'm just slowing up here."

When eleven days had gone by I took the home pregnancy test, and it was positive. Since I hadn't had any spotting at all, when I saw the positive result I actually allowed myself to hope. Something inside me said, "Maybe there's a chance for this one."

That was a Sunday and I went to church the way I always do. That day in church I really prayed for a baby for the first time. The other times I'd pray and say, "If you think I deserve it, fine." But this time I prayed to Mary and I said, "Look, you're a mother. Help me have this one. If you do I'll name the baby after you."

The next day I called my doctor and he said to come in. I was going to, but then I changed my mind. Something inside me snapped. I finally realized that I hadn't been getting the best medical care that I could have been getting and I thought, "I can't go through another pregnancy with this doctor. He's not equipped to handle my problem."

I called Robert Wood Johnson Hospital, which is in New Brunswick near where I live and is associated with the University of Medicine and Dentistry in New Jersey. Because of my job selling laboratory equipment and supplies, I had recently started selling to Robert Wood Johnson and realized it was a very good hospital, and that they would refer me to a good doctor. The person I spoke with gave me the names of two groups of doctors.

I called both. At this point I was desperate. I knew I was pregnant, and for the first time in years I actually thought this pregnancy stood a chance. I was determined to get somewhere this time. If the doctor didn't seem like he really knew what he was doing, I wasn't going to see him. I was just determined to get someone who was going to help me.

One group of doctors called me back. I explained my situation and they said there was only one group in all of Central Jersey that could help me. It was associated with St. Peter's Medical Center, which handles high-risk pregnancies and is also associated with the University of Medicine and Dentistry in New Jersey. This was the second group the person at Robert Wood Johnson had recommended, the group that hadn't called me back.

When I'd called the group at St. Peter's I'd told whoever answered the phone how desperate I was to see a doctor. I'd made it clear that I needed a call back that day, and when they didn't call me back I was a wreck. I felt that with every minute that passed I was running the risk of losing the baby if I was not doing something that I should be doing, so when I didn't get a call back I said, "I'm not going to put up with this."

At six o'clock that evening I called them again. The office was closed, and I had them page the doctor on call. Dr. Chris Houlihan called me back, and before he could stop me I blurted out my story. It took twenty minutes to tell him everything. I let him know how desperate I was, how determined. I said, "I'm pregnant now. I really need to have someone good to help me."

His answer was, "Oh wow." Then he said, "Why don't you come in tomorrow?" I couldn't believe it because usually you have to wait a very long time to see doctors who are this good.

I went in the next day. I didn't learn until I went in that Dr. Houlihan was a very young doctor who was out of residency maybe a year or two and was completing his fellowship in high-risk pregnancies. If they accepted me as a patient, Dr. Edwin Guzman would actually be my physician. I could hear Dr. Guzman in the doctor's area giving Dr. Houlihan hell for having me come in. He was saying, "We are here to help the patients of other doctors, not to take away patients of other doctors. You can't just have a patient walk in. This woman's doctor should have called us." To me, he seemed to be saying, "I'm going to get rid of her."

When Dr. Guzman walked in to see me I was a wreck. I told him my story, and he said the thing that impressed him about me was that I was a great historian. I was able to tell him exactly what had happened to me and when. I had brought a file with me that had all the dates of my pregnancies and the dates those pregnancies ended. I had all my test results, all my numbers. It was just my nature, as I was going along with all my pregnancies, to write everything down. I kept as much information as I could.

He saw I wasn't kidding, that I'd been through a lot of doctors and that now I really wanted to go to someone who could help me. He said, "As long as your doctor releases you I will take you as a patient." He called my doctor who said, "Well, you know I can handle her," and Dr. Guzman said, "Yes I know you can but she came to us and she would like to be our patient now." And so my doctor released me.

It turned out that all the neurological symptoms I had experienced are ones that can occur with my condition. I learned that when you have this condition, you should keep on top of it with a rheumatologist.* No doctor had ever told me this before, and I

---

* A rheumotologist specializes in autoimmune diseases which is what APLS falls under. The neurologic symptoms are *one* manifestation of the disease.

hadn't seen anything in my own research saying my condition could cause problems for the mother.

Dr. Guzman told me I should go on aspirin right away. I was reluctant to tell them I was on aspirin already, but once I'd explained what I'd been doing, they said to continue to take the aspirin and that later on they would start me on heparin, which is a stronger blood thinner than aspirin. I asked if I'd have to take prednisone, but they said it wasn't necessary, that aspirin and heparin would be enough for me.

Soon I started spotting, and I bled through the rest of my first three months. The bleeding was a very heavy black discharge. Though they said it was implantation bleeding, I felt they didn't really know what was causing it because they said, "We're going to keep going on, and as long as you're not losing the pregnancy we've got hope."

I was threatening to miscarry, but they didn't want to tell me that. I called them constantly, and they kept reassuring me that everything was going to be fine. Every two weeks they did an ultrasound on me, and the baby continued developing well.

I got to three months, and they started me on heparin. I had to give myself injections of it twice a day. After the third injection I was in the shower and passed two huge blood clots—the size of the palm of your hand. I was bleeding all over the place, in the tub, on the floor. It was a mess. I thought for sure I was losing the baby. I called the doctor, and he had me come in immediately.

I could see the concern on their faces when they

walked into the examining room. They were very quiet. I was shaking. John was with me, and before they started the ultrasound they said, "Be prepared." And we were.

The doctors would always look at the screen together and start pointing things out. They did the same thing this time. They said, "This looks good and that looks good. The heartbeat's there and this looks good." Then they started using medical terms, and I knew that everything was all right. When the ultrasound was done, Dr. Guzman said, "Karen, you've given me a heart attack here. Why did you do this to me? Everything's fine." Of course I was relieved, but the emotional swing was hard. I had been down so low, and I had to come right back up again.

The doctors said the heparin didn't cause the blood clots to pass, but they can't convince me of that. I'm convinced that blood clots were starting to form and, had I not started taking heparin, the aspirin alone would not have been the answer for me. But they felt the blood clots were probably just something that happened.

The next day I stopped bleeding and never bled a drop again. But I never stopped worrying. I saw the doctors every two weeks. They'd both see me, and they'd check me and the progress of the baby and the circulation of blood to the uterus and the placenta with an ultrasound. Before each visit I'd sit in the waiting room, terrified that I wouldn't hear a heartbeat. I'd think, "Please, let me hear that sound." Because when you don't hear it—when there's that dead silence—it's so awful. Just so awful.

But at each visit I heard the heartbeat. The pregnancy progressed. I started having contractions at around the twelfth week. Every time I got in the car and drove I felt them, but when I was walking around they would subside. At around the seventeenth week my cervix began dilating. They watched me and at the nineteenth week they said, "We have to do a cerclage."

They put in a cervical stitch and asked if I wanted to go on bed rest because of the contractions and my cervix. I took a week off but couldn't stand being home and said, "If it's not going to cause me a problem I would like to continue working."

And so I did. By this time the amnio results had come back normal and revealed that I was carrying a girl. At the twenty-sixth week I started having some heavy contractions, and they said I had to stop working. At about the thirtieth week just sitting would cause me to have contractions, so I had to lie down most of the day. They were afraid the stitch would go, but it didn't.

They took the stitch out in the thirty-sixth week. They thought I would give birth that night, but I went another four weeks. I carried her to term. She was due on the eleventh, and she came on the tenth.

During the entire pregnancy I never, ever thought that I would have a baby. I couldn't even imagine it. I had come to associate pregnancy with loss. Whenever someone told me she was pregnant I would look at her and think, "My God, you don't know what you're in for. You're going to be devastated when you lose that pregnancy." I would see some really happy pregnant women and I would want to tell them, "Don't get too excited, kiddo, because you could lose it." When some of them miscarried, I would think, "See, you shouldn't have allowed yourself to get that happy." When their pregnancies actually resulted in a baby, I would be amazed.

Even when I was up on the table giving birth I couldn't imagine that I would have a living being to bring home. I was convinced that something was going to go wrong, so I didn't bond with the baby when she was inside me. But once she was born and I heard her cry, that was it for me. We were buddies.

I feel really lucky that I found Houlihan and Guzman. They had all the right ingredients for me. I sensed immediately that they knew what they were doing. They took the time with me in the beginning to understand what was going on with me. They explained a lot more to me than any other doctor had. They assured me that they could help me. Their nurses assured me that they could help me. They were confident they could handle the problem. I never doubted them even though the method of treatment for my condition is still trial and error. Even though they disagreed sometimes, I always felt that, in the end, they made an informed decision. They also referred me to a rheumatologist who told me that I will need to take aspirin every day for the rest of my life. I see him every six months.

I don't know—and the doctors said they didn't know—why my taking the low-dose aspirin for two months while I was pregnant with Allison worked, and why my being on aspirin and prednisone during the previous normal pregnancy didn't. I think it's because my condition is cyclical; there are times when the antibody count can be very high and times when it can be lower.

I remembered the promise I'd made when I prayed for this baby, and I named my daughter Allison Marie. When I gave birth to Allison I was 41. I quit work and will stay home with her until she goes to school. I will not have another baby. It's not recommended for me because heparin takes a toll on your body, and when you take it your chances of osteoporosis are greatly increased.

Having Allison is a nice ending to a long battle. She's eased some of the pain that I've felt over the years, but the pain of the stillbirth is something I'll never get over. Nothing could ease that pain. I do think, however, that a support group or a therapist could have helped. At the time, I thought I had to work through it myself but, looking back, I don't think that's the best thing to do. When you hold your grief in and try to go on with life as usual, life is never usual for you. The grief is always with you and will linger a lot longer than you realize.

Finally, I would say to anyone who is suffering pregnancy losses the way I did, "Don't give up hope." Adoption is great if that feels right for you, but remember that breakthroughs are right around the corner. The answers to my problem came into true focus only very recently, and doctors are learning more about how to treat it every day. There's a lot of research going on and maybe, one day, that research will hold the answer for you.

ANONYMOUS
NUMBER OF MISCARRIAGES: FIVE KNOWN
CAUSE: UNKNOWN. ASSUMED TO BE IMMUNOLOGICAL

For ten long, desperate years my husband and I tried to have a baby. It would take me a long time to conceive—first naturally and later through in vitro fertilization—and then I would miscarry. That happened five times.

When I say those years were desperate, I mean *desperate*. We tried everything—all sorts of doctors here and abroad, but none of them could ever tell me what was causing my miscarriages. Although I never had an official diagnosis, I took progesterone, baby aspirin, prednisone, and heparin—all at the same time—"just in case" those medications could correct whatever was going wrong in my body. I had my husband's white blood cells injected into me "just in case" I wasn't making fetal-blocking antibodies. I even wore a monitor that was supposed to purge my body of all its toxins.

Nothing worked, but still I wouldn't give up. I'd conceived my last pregnancy through in vitro fertilization, and I was all set to go through in vitro again when I got a phone call. Someone in our community knew a woman who was pregnant and wanted to put the child up for adoption.

My immediate reaction was no. When I called my husband to tell him I'd gotten this phone call he said, "Just say no," and he hung up the phone. We didn't take it seriously, but then I started thinking about how rare it was to get an opportunity like this.

A baby was being handed to me like a present wrapped in a bow. That night, I said to my husband, "You know, maybe we should think about this."

We had to make a decision quickly, and that week we went four times to see a therapist to help us decide what to do. The therapist asked me to write down all the reasons I didn't want to adopt, and I filled up a sheet of yellow legal paper in two minutes. The first thing I wrote was, "I got an F on my report card."

I saw adoption as a failure and that was the biggest thing stopping me. My husband and I are both goody-two-shoes. We are successful attorneys who worked hard to get to where we are in life. Even though we had these awful obstacles to conquer when it came to having children, we believed that if we tried hard enough we would conquer them. Adopting a baby would mean I hadn't succeeded in what I had tried to do, and that close to ten years of trying and researching and seeing doctors would be thrown out. I felt like I would have gone through all that pain for nothing, and I wasn't ready to give up the fight. I miscarried my first pregnancy in 1986. It was a blighted ovum, which means there was a sac but no embryo. My husband and I were very upset, but everyone minimized our loss. My doctor said, "It's no big deal. Everyone miscarries." I kept my miscarriage from most people, but those who knew said really insensitive things like, "It's for the best. The baby would have been mentally retarded." No one understood the emotional pain my husband and I were going through.

I didn't get pregnant again for another two years, so I went to see a few fertility doctors, none of whom could find any reason for my infertility. When I finally did get pregnant again, the embryo never developed a heartbeat.

The doctors did genetic testing on the embryo, but everything came back normal. My husband and I went for extensive testing, and those results all came back normal, too. But the doctor said the next time I got pregnant he would put me on progesterone "just in case" I was having some sort of progesterone defect.

The same thing that had happened with my second pregnancy happened with my third. My numbers (HCG and progesterone levels) started to drop in the fifth week, the baby never developed a heartbeat, and I had a D&C at eight weeks.

After that miscarriage the doctor said, "Let's not take any chances. Let's put you on baby aspirin just in case." Because he could find no reason for my miscarriages, he said the cause was probably immunological. The field of immunology is where doctors' knowledge is the weakest and they have the least data. My doctor—and all the other doctors I saw—categorized me in that area for lack of anything else.

After my third miscarriage, all hell broke loose. The genetic testing on that baby came back normal, too, so it was clear that something was definitely going on in my body. That's when my doctor told me about Dr. Cowchock and Dr. Beer who, separately, were conducting research on women who weren't producing the fetal-blocking antibodies you need in

order to protect your pregnancy. (For more information on Dr. F. Susan Cowchock and Dr. Alan Beer and
their research on fetal-blocking antibody deficiency,
see Chapter 4 and Appendix I.) Dr. Beer in Chicago
accepted me into his program and injected me with
my husband's white blood cells.

The pregnancy after that treatment made it to ten
weeks. For the first time I got to see a heartbeat—not
just once, but on three different sonograms. We felt
sure that we had conquered our problem, and what a
wonderful feeling that was!

I saw the heartbeat on the third sonogram on a
Thursday; the following Monday it was gone. That
was my fourth loss, and that was the worst. I was destroyed. It was the worst day of my life. I remember
very desperately wanting to jump off a bridge.

For that pregnancy I had gone to Dr. Beer and had
also been on baby aspirin, heparin, prednisone, and
progesterone. I was a walking pharmacy. I was fat,
ugly, full of pimples, and bloated, and the prednisone was making me nuts. I had been on a very
high dose—50 mgs a day—and when I lost the baby
no one was smart enough to tell me to wean myself
off it. I went cold turkey, and first my knees and then
all of my joints locked. It was awful. But what I went
through physically was nothing compared to what I
went through emotionally.

The week after the miscarriage I couldn't sleep. I
spent the nights writing and writing even though I
hate to write. I would write about how I hated everyone and everything. I let my anger out that way. One
of the things that I wrote was a letter to the support

group RESOLVE. I wanted to know whether anyone else had experienced repeated miscarriages that were unexplained. I was the only person I knew who was going through this.

One woman told me she'd gone through it for seventeen years and then finally had a baby after being treated for fetal-blocking antibody deficiency by Dr. Cowchock. But I'd already tried that treatment with Dr. Beer, and it hadn't worked for me.

Another woman told me about a doctor in New York who does research on toxic bacteria. Half the doctors thought he was the biggest quack in town, but I was desperate. I didn't have the luxury not to believe what he was doing, because the doctors who had the best reputation were saying to me, "We don't know what to do with you." My own doctor, who's a well-known fertility expert, is a real optimist. He'd always told me not to worry, that there was hope for me, but he threw up his hands after my fourth loss.

I went to this doctor who was doing research on bacteria that might be toxic to the fetus. He had me and my husband wear bacteria monitors for a week to try to kill off all the potentially toxic bacteria in our bodies.

Besides wearing the monitor, I decided I was going to try the in vitro fertilization programs to try to speed the process along. The IVF experts told me they couldn't take me into their programs because I was getting pregnant. I said, "Yes. But I keep miscarrying. Maybe the fact that I have a hard time conceiving has something to do with the miscarriages." (To this day the doctors are convinced that there was some link between the two, but they don't know what that link is. They say I probably had more miscarriages than I even know about, but that those pregnancies weren't documented.)

I really tried to talk my way into the IVF programs. I would say, "I know I'm conceiving, but it takes me such a long time and now I'm over thirty. I could have ten more miscarriages. I don't know how long this is going to take, and if I can better my odds of having a successful pregnancy by getting pregnant more often I'll do it."

One of the reasons I hated miscarrying was because that meant that for the next two months I couldn't try conceiving. To me that was the worst. Even if the pregnancy didn't work at least I'd know I'd tried. If I couldn't try I was nuts. I always tried to conceive as soon as I could, and now I wanted to conceive as much as I could. A doctor at one of the IVF programs said, "You're not a candidate for us, but I'm sure you have scar tissue from all the D&Cs you had because of your miscarriages." I said I'd had hysterosalpingograms twice, but he convinced me to have one again. It showed that everything was fine. Afterward, he felt so bad for me that he let me come into his IVF program. He let me in out of pity, which was awful. If you're used to being successful and to being perceived as a success, it's terrible to have people look at you with pity.

I'm Orthodox and I come from a society and a neighborhood where people have six or eight or ten kids without blinking. I have two sisters; one of them has six kids and the other has four. They both had their kids very easily. Their hearts cried for me when I miscarried. I'm very close with them, but it wasn't easy for me when they called to tell me they were pregnant. Does that mean I'm a horrible person? I don't know. That's how it felt. It hurt. It hurt like hell.

I tried to keep my miscarriages a secret from everyone but my family, and even today I don't tell people about what I went through. I know that my miscarriages were out of my control, yet to me, the fact that I kept miscarrying is something I'm embarrassed about. It's a stigma on me. If I think logically that's like saying if someone has cancer then they have a stigma on them, and I know that's not true. But, still, that's how I feel about my miscarriages.

Even though I tried to keep my miscarriages a secret, people in my community guessed that I was having some sort of trouble getting pregnant. Strangers would come over to me and say, "Don't worry, darling you'll have children." They would offer to give me the name of a person who had helped them. They were trying to be sweet, and if I was in a good mood their efforts to help me wouldn't bother me. But if I was having a bad day I'd want to say to those people, "Who asked you? I don't even know who you are. Why are you delving into my personal life?" It was no one's business if I didn't have kids because I was miscarrying or because I just couldn't get pregnant. People really didn't hesitate to ask me what the problem was, even though this was something I clearly didn't want to share with anyone. I thought they were invading my bedroom.

Even though I was trying to keep things a secret, there were some pretty visible signs of what I was going through, namely the stunning black-and-blue marks I would have from injecting myself with heparin. Even though I'd worn the bacteria monitor, I was still continuing all my other treatments as I tried to get pregnant again. This time my doctor said that instead of starting the heparin after I was pregnant, I should start it postovulation. That was awful because I was stabbing myself twice a day, I wasn't even pregnant, and I'd have those black-and-blue marks. It sounds like a stupid thing to be concerned about, but if it's summer you can't go out in a bathing suit. When you go in to try on a dress in a clothing store the saleswoman stares at you. If you're traveling, you need a letter from your doctor saying that you can have needles on the plane, or else airport security will stop you. None of this was insurmountable, but it was a visible, daily reminder to myself and everyone else of what I was going through, and it didn't pay off.

My fifth pregnancy was a chemical pregnancy. As soon as he gave me the numbers my doctor said, "This pregnancy won't last. It's too low." Emotionally, the fifth miscarriage was the least devastating because as soon as they gave me the news they said that it wasn't going to last. The fifth one was the only one I didn't need a D&C for. It bled out. That's also better because you don't have to go through a surgical procedure.

A few months after this miscarriage was when the adoption was presented to me. My doctor was all for the adoption. He said, "Even if you have a baby someday, I think you have enough love to go around. So what if you have another one. And you know what? It will probably ease the pressure you're feeling to have a baby. In case you have a lot more miscarriages they will be easier deal with if you have a baby at home." My sisters were great, too. They said, "You love our kids. You're going to love this one, too."

But I wasn't convinced. My list of negatives included, "I'm afraid of not loving the baby enough" and "I'm afraid that other people in the family won't love the baby enough" and "What if I do give birth to a baby? What will it be like having two different kinds of babies?"

But the biggest thing in my mind was that I really did see it as a failure. Despite all that, we decided to take the baby because the opportunity was unbelievably great. All you need to do is talk to people who want to adopt, and they'll tell you about how difficult it is. I didn't know if opportunity would knock again. I knew I wasn't going to give up my pursuit of having my own child, but who knew if I would ever be successful?

My doctor couldn't understand why I wanted my own child so much, but I wanted the experience of having my own child. I didn't understand that when you adopt a child, you don't love him any differently than a child you give birth to.

How do I know that? Because nineteen months after I adopted, I gave birth to a baby boy. Now, because I do have one of each kind I can say, "There is no difference."

No one knows how I finally came to give birth. You hear these stories about how after people adopt they conceive because the stress is off, and maybe that's what happened. I still wanted to give birth to my own baby and I thought I was stressed about it, but maybe on some level the stress was eased a bit because we had adopted this baby who was the greatest thing in the world.

When I conceived it was through an IVF program. I had eighteen eggs and only one fertilized. I remember saying to the doctor, *"One?* Boy is this a waste of time." But he said, "It's a really good one." In my mind I dismissed the pregnancy. I remember that on the night I heard that I was borderline positive I went out and had a drink. With all the previous pregnancies, the minute I heard I was pregnant I wouldn't touch a drop of alcohol. But I was thought, "Naaah, not this time."

A few days later, my HCG level doubled the way it was supposed to, and that was when I started to do everything possible to make the pregnancy work. I flew to Chicago for a boost to my fetal-blocking antibodies, just in case that treatment did work. I went on every medication again—baby aspirin, heparin, prednisone, and progesterone injections.

It was a very very difficult pregnancy, especially the first ten weeks because all my other pregnancies had ended before then. Getting past the hurdle of six weeks was significant. Getting past the hurdle of eight weeks was major. Getting past the hurdle of ten weeks was beyond belief. In my seventeenth week they discharged me to a high-risk pregnancy doctor.

That week, I started falling to the floor and no one knew why. The first day it happened I went to work. The second day every time I tried to hold my blow-dryer and get dressed, I couldn't. I went to the obstetrician who said, "The baby's fine. Maybe you have an ear infection." He gave me the name of an internist, and he said, "You're losing all your blood. Something's going wrong. Go get a blood transfusion right now."

It turned out that the blood thinners had thinned my blood to a point that was causing internal bleeding. They gave me three blood transfusions and told me I had to stop all my medications. I was shrieking. I was terrified that I would lose the pregnancy, but they said my life was at stake. I had to stop.

I was sure I would lose the pregnancy, but the placenta held its own. The baby was born two months early, and now I have two wonderful little boys.

I know this is going to sound ridiculous, but I believe that the child we adopted was meant to come to our home. Had we not gone through our miscarriages, he obviously wouldn't be here. I know that sounds crazy, but I'm convinced that's the only way he could have been raised in our home, and that's why we had to go through this.

Now I have a lot of couples come to me when they start thinking about adoption, and they ask me if I was scared of adopting our son. I remind myself of that legal pad. Scared isn't the word, but adopting him was the best decision we ever made. He's the greatest most wonderful kid, and I love him just as if he was my own, because he is.

EPILOGUE

Just as everyone's experience with miscarriage is unique, so too is everyone's resolution of the pain they felt over their miscarriage or miscarriages. Most parents say their grief feels fully resolved only after they have children, either through childbirth or through adoption. Those who miscarry repeatedly yet decide not to adopt say their pain lessens only after they've made a final decision not to have children and have stopped trying and have moved on with their lives.

Whatever your miscarriage story and your final outcome, the most important thing you can do is move on with your life, too. This is something that will happen naturally with time. Time, after all, is indeed a great healer. Know that your pain over your loss will never fully go away, but it will move into a different place in your heart and mind. We hope this book has helped it get there.

Appendix I

▼

RESOURCES

SUPPORT GROUPS

SHARE—Pregnancy and Infant Loss Support, Inc
St. Joseph Health Center
300 First Capitol Drive
St. Charles, MO 63301-893
(800) 821-6819
http://www.nationalshareoffice.com

This is the national office for a network of support groups across the United States and Canada. They will send you, free of charge, a packet of information about the emotional side of miscarriage and also a list of support groups in your state. They also publish a bimonthly newsletter featuring writings by couples who have experienced miscarriage or stillbirth, as well as informative articles on those subjects. A subscription is free for the first year.

NATIONAL RESOLVE
1310 Broadway, Dept. GM
Somerville, MA 02144-1731
(617) 623-0744
http://www.resolve.org

This is a support group primarily for infertile women, but they can also put you in touch with women who have suffered recurrent miscarriages.

Pregnancy and Infant Loss Center
1421 East Wayzata Boulevard
Wayzata, MN 55391
(612) 473-9372
http://www.bloomington.in.us/socserv/mit/pregnancy-and-infant-loss-center.html

Provides nationwide referrals to support groups for people who have suffered miscarriage, stillbirth, and infant death. You can request a catalogue of books and also a copy of their quarterly newsletter dealing with the emotional side of coping with pregnancy loss. The catalogue and one issue of the newsletter will be sent to you free of charge. An annual subscription to the newsletter costs $20.

INFORMATION ON THE TREATMENT OF FETAL-BLOCKING ANTIBODY DEFICIENCY

Dr. F. Susan Cowchock
Professor of Obstetrics and Gynecology
Director, Recurrent Pregnancy Loss Program
New York University Medical Center
550 First Avenue
New York, NY 10016
(212) 263-1060

Dr. Alan E. Beer
Director of Reproductive Medicine
Finch University of Health Sciences/
The Chicago Medical School
3333 Green Bay Road
North Chicago, IL 60064
(708) 578-3233

Appendix II

▼

FURTHER READING

BOOKS ON MISCARRIAGE

Your local bookstore can order any of the following for you:

Allen, Marie, and Shelly Marks. *Miscarriage: Women Sharing from the Heart.* New York: Wiley, 1993.

Kohn, Ingrid, and Perry-Lynn Moffitt. *A Silent Sorrow: Pregnancy Loss.* New York: Dell, 1992.

Pizer, Hank, and Christine O. Palinski. *Coping with a Miscarriage.* New York: NAL-Dutton, 1986.

Scher, Jonathan, and Carol Dix. *Preventing a Miscarriage: The Good News.* New York: Harper Collins, 1991.

Senchyshyn, Stefan, and Carol Colman. *How to Prevent Miscarriage and Other Crises of Pregnancy.* New York: Macmillan, 1990.

BOOKS ON GRIEVING A LOSS

Bozarth, Alla Renee, Ph.D. *Life Is Goodbye, Life Is Hello: Grieving Well Through All Kinds of Loss.* Minnesota: Hazelden, 1986.

Bramblett, John. *When Good-bye Is Forever: Learning to Live Again After the Loss of a Child.* New York: Ballantine, 1991.

Crenshaw, David A., Ph.D. *Bereavement: Counseling the Grieving Throughout the Life Cycle.* New York: Crossroad, 1995.

Fitzgerald, Helen. *The Mourning Handbook.* New York: Simon & Schuster, 1994.

Kübler-Ross, Elisabeth. *On Death and Dying.* New York: Collier Books/Macmillan, 1993.

Woodson, Meg. *Making It Through the Toughest Days of Grief: Anniversaries, Holidays and Other Landmark Days.* New York: Harper Paperbacks, 1994.

GLOSSARY

Abortion: Though commonly used to refer to an elective procedure undergone to terminate an unwanted pregnancy, in medical terminology the word refers to the loss of a pregnancy, no matter what its cause.

Accutane: A drug prescribed for severe acne, it can seriously harm a fetus. Any woman who has taken it should have stopped doing so for at least six months before becoming pregnant to ensure that the drug is out of her system.

Antiphospholipid syndrome (APLS): An autoimmune syndrome. Those with autoimmune syndromes produce antibodies to their own tissues or cells; these are called *autoantibodies*. Those with APLS produce autoantibodies to phospholipids, fatty molecules on the cell membranes. These autoantibodies cause blood clots to form in various parts of the body; if they form in the placenta, the fetus will be deprived of oxygen and nutrients. Unfortunately, the main symptom of APLS is recurrent pregnancy loss (APLS acounts for 10 to 15 percent of recurrent miscarriages); once suspected, it can be diagnosed through blood tests.

Cervix: The neck, or narrow part, of the uterus that protrudes into the vaginal cavity.

Chromosomal abnormalities: Errors in chromosomal division that result in invalid coding, or instructions, for embryonic growth, thereby making the pregnancy nonviable or abnormal. These random errors cannot be anticipated, treated, or prevented; they are the cause of 50 to 60 percent of all miscarriages.

Chromosome: Any of the microscopic rod-shaped bodies in the cell nucleus which separates during mitosis, or division; chromosomes carry the genes, which convey hereditary characteristics.

Conception: The fertilization of an egg by sperm, resulting in pregnancy.

Corpus luteum: The small yellow structure that forms in the ovary following release of the egg (ovulation) from the ruptured ovarian follicle; it produces the hormone progesterone, responsible for counteracting the build-up of estrogen in the uterine lining during the second half of the menstrual cycle, and it supports a newly formed pregnancy.

Cytomegalovirus: An infection harmful to pregnancy, it is a flulike virus common in children.

Death in utero: The loss of a developing pregnancy after the twentieth week following the last menstrual period.

Diethylstilbestrol (DES): A synthetic hormone first commonly prescribed in 1949 and finally made illegal in 1971; ironically, it was prescribed to prevent miscarriage, but has caused fusion defects (uterine abnormalities) in many of the daughters of women who took it, causing them to miscarry.

Dilatation and curettage (D&C): A surgical procedure in which the cervix is dilated and the lining of the uterus is scraped with a curette, a sharp instrument that looks like a hollow spoon.

Ectopic pregnancy: A pregnancy in which the fertilized egg (zygote) implants outside the uterus. Types of ectopic pregnancy are abdominal pregnancy, ovarian pregnancy, and tubal pregnancy, in which the egg implants in one of the fallopian tubes. An ectopic pregnancy is diagnosed by a sonogram; it cannot be carried to term. Ninety-five percent of ectopic pregnancies are in the fallopian tubes.

Embryo: Once the fertilized egg (the zygote) has attached itself to the lining of the uterus (the endometrium), and the placenta begins to grow, the pregnancy is now referred to as an embryo; after the embryo has developed for twelve weeks, it is referred to as a fetus.

Endometrium: The lining of the internal surface of the uterus into which the fertilized egg (zygote) implants; if conception has not occurred, the endometrium is shed during menstruation.

Fallopian tubes: Long, slender tubes extending from each side of the uterus and ending near the ovaries; fertilization normally occurs within these tubes.

Fetal-blocking antibodies: Proteins created by the mother's body to protect the pregnancy from her other antibodies, which would otherwise recognize the pregnancy as foreign and reject it.

Fetus: The developing pregnancy from twelve weeks until birth.

Fibroid: A benign tumor of the uterus consisting of fibrous and muscle tissue.

Follicle stimulating hormone (FSH): A hormone secreted by the pituitary gland that stimulates the growth of egg sacs (follicles) in the ovaries.

Fusion defect: An anatomic defect in which the uterus, cervix, or upper vagina did not fuse completely or properly; also called a *uterine abnormality or anomaly.*

Gonadotropin releasing hormone (GnRH): A hormone produced by the hypothalamus; it stimulates the pituitary gland to produce both follicle stimulating hormone (FSH) and luteinizing hormone (LH).

Habitual aborter: The medical term for a woman who has suffered three consecutive miscarriages due to an underlying condition that must be treated before she will be able to carry to term; also called *recurrent aborter.*

Habitual abortion workup: Series of medical tests performed to determine if an underlying recurring problem is causing consecutive miscarriages. Formerly, such a workup was not performed until a woman had had three consecutive miscarriages; nowadays, with so many women conceiving later in life, the workup is performed after two consecutive miscarriages.

Heparin: The drug heparin sodium, used to prevent blood clotting; it is used to treat antiphospholipid syndrome.

Herpes: An infection harmful to pregnancy. Type 1 is most commonly seen in oral infections, Type 2 most commonly in genital infections; it is caused by skin-to-skin contact with someone who has herpes lesions.

Human chorionic gonadotropin (HCG): Hormone released by cells in the placenta; it causes the fertilized egg to release estrogen and progesterone. Home pregnancy tests screen for it; it is also what doctors look for in blood tests to confirm pregnancy.

Hypothalamus: The part of the brain that controls the glandular (endocrine) system. Among the hormones secreted by the hypothalamus is gonadotropin releasing hormone (GnRH).

Hysterosalpingogram: A diagnostic medical test made to determine if a woman has a septate uterus. *See* Septate uterus *and* Septum.

Hysteroscopic resection: A surgical procedure performed to correct certain intrauterine abnormalities, including a septate uterus. After using a fiber-optic scope to determine the location of the septum in the uterus, the doctor inserts a sharp instrument called a resectoscope into the uterus to shave off the septum and create a near normal uterine cavity. *See* Septate uterus *and* Septum.

IgG: Immunoglobulin; an antibody produced to fight an infection. Once produced, some level of it will remain in the blood throughout a person's lifetime.

IgM: Immunoglobulin; an antibody present only during the acute phase of an infection.

Incompetent cervix: A cervix that is too weak to support the increased pressure of a growing pregnancy.

Luteal phase defect (LPD): A condition in which a woman does not produce enough progesterone to properly prepare her endometrial lining to accept a fertilized egg for implantation. Sometimes women who believe they are infertile are actually conceiving but, due to LPD, are miscarrying at a very early stage.

Luteinizing hormone (LH): A hormone secreted by the pituitary gland that stimulates the ripening and release of an egg from the ovaries.

Miscarriage: The loss of a developing pregnancy at any time from conception until the twentieth week after the last menstrual period.

Monosomy: A chromosomal error in which the fertilized egg has only one chromosome where there should have been a pair.

Non-disjunction: The most frequently occurring chromosomal error; the chromosomes in the egg split unevenly during either the egg's first division, when it is getting ready to be released (to be ovulated), or during the second division, when it is being fertilized.

Oocyte: Egg; prior to its first chromosomal division, it is termed a primary oocyte; after its first chromosomal division, it is termed a secondary oocyte.

Ovary: The female reproductive gland (there are two of them) that produces eggs and the sex hormones estrogen and progesterone.

Ovulation: The monthly release of an egg by the ovaries.

Placenta: An organ that develops within the uterus during pregnancy to deliver nourishment to the fetus, to which it is connected by the umbilical cord.

Prenatal: Before birth.

Progesterone: A hormone produced by the corpus luteum after a woman ovulates; it prepares the endometrium for pregnancy. A fall in progesterone production initiates the menstrual period.

Random chromosomal error: *See* Chromosomal abnormalities.

Random miscarriage: The isolated loss of a pregnancy due most often to a nonrecurring chromosomal error or other problem in the fetus.

Recurrent aborter: *See* Habitual aborter.

Recurring miscarriage: The habitual loss of pregnancy due to some underlying condition that will generally need to be treated before the woman will be able to carry to term; 20 percent of women who miscarry will become what are referrred to in medical terminology as *habitual* or *recurrent* aborters.

Rubella: Long known as German measles; an infection harmful to pregnancy; transmitted during respiration in the presence of an infected individual.

Septate uterus: A mild fusion defect that occurred when the uterus was being formed. A fibrous membrane called a septum extends into the uterus at the point where the fusion did not occur properly. Since the septum has few blood vessels, it inhibits the growth of the placenta in that region, which could cause miscarriage. *See* Septum.

Septum: A fibrous membrane that extends into the uterus at the point where fusion did not occur properly when the uterus was being formed. *See* Septate uterus.

Sonogram: The process of imaging deep structures of the body by recording the reflection of high-frequency sound waves; among its uses are the diagnosis of fetal abnormalities. Also known as *ultrasound*.

Sporadic miscarriage: *See* Random miscarriage.

Tetraploidy: A chromosomal error in which the fertilized egg has 92 chromosomes (it should have 46); either three sperm fertilized the egg, or two eggs and two sperm somehow merged. Ten percent of all first trimester miscarriages that are caused by chromosomal error are tetraploidies.

Titer: The measuring unit used when blood is screened for antibodies to viral infections.

Toxoplasmosis: An infection harmful to pregnancy; caused by a parasite carried in infected cat feces and undercooked meat or fish.

Triploidy: A chromosomal error in which the fertilized egg has a chromosomal count of 69 (it should be 46); it is generally believed that this error results when two sperm fertilize an egg. Twenty percent of all first trimester miscarriages that are caused by chromosomal error are triploidies.

Trisomy: A chromosomal error in which a fertilized egg will have one chromosome too many somewhere along its lineup of 23 chromosomal pairs. Fifty percent of all first trimester miscarriages that are caused by chromosomal error are trisomies.

Uterine abnormality: *See* Fusion defect.

Uterus: The thick-walled muscular cavity within a woman's pelvis that contains and nourishes a growing fetus during pregnancy.

Vagina: The canal extending from the vulva to the cervix.

Vulva: Woman's external genital organs, including the mons pubis, labia majora, labia minora, clitoris, and other structures.

INDEX

ABOUT THE AUTHORS

LYNN FRIEDMAN, M.D., is an assistant clinical professor at Mount Sinai Medical Center in New York City. She attended New York University Medical School and completed her internship and residency in obstetrics and gynecology at Mount Sinai Medical Center.

IRENE DARIA is an award-winning, multifaceted writer and editor. She is the former health editor of *Woman's World,* where she is currently special features editor. She is the author of two other books: *The Fashion Cycle* and *Lutèce: A Day in the Life of America's Greatest Restaurant.* She has worked as a reporter at *Women's Wear Daily* and as an editor at *Harper's Bazaar,* and her articles have appeared in the *New York Times, Money, Glamour, Mademoiselle,* and many other publications.

Look for these other titles in the Woman Doctor's Series from Kensington Publishing:

Menopause: A Woman Doctor's Guide
by
Lois Jovanovic, M.D. with Suzanne LeVert

PMS: A Woman Doctor's Guide
by
Andrea J. Rapkin, M.D., FACOG, with Diana Tonnessen

Infertility: A Woman Doctor's Guide
by
Susan Treiser, M.D., with Robin K. Levinson

Skin Care: A Woman Doctor's Guide
by
Wilma F. Bergfeld, M.D., with Shelagh Ryan Masline

Osteoporosis: A Woman Doctor's Guide
by
Yvonne, R. Sherrer, M.D., with Robin K. Levinson